The Epidemiology and Prevention of Important Diseases

The Epidemiology and Prevention of Important Diseases

I D Gerald Richards MD PhD FRCP FFCM DPH
Professor of Community Medicine, University of Leeds

Mark R Baker MD MSc MRCP FFCM
District General Manager, Bradford Health Authority; Honorary Professor of Public Health and
Director of the Clinical Epidemiology Research Unit, University of Bradford

CHURCHILL LIVINGSTONE
EDINBURGH LONDON MELBOURNE AND NEW YORK 1988

CHURCHILL LIVINGSTONE
Medical Division of Longman Group UK Limited

Distributed in the United States of America by Churchill
Livingstone Inc., 1560 Broadway, New York, N.Y.
10036, and by associated companies, branches and
representatives throughout the world.

First published 1988

ISBN 0-443-02587-8

British Library Cataloguing in Publication Data
Richards, I. D. Gerald.
  The epidemiology and prevention of
  important diseases
  1. Epidemiology
  I. Title II. Baker, Mark R.
  614.4 RA651

Library of Congress Cataloging in Publication Data
Richards, I. D. Gerald.
  The epidemiology and prevention of important
diseases.
  Includes index.
  1. Epidemiology. 2. Medicine, Preventive. I. Baker,
Mark R. II. Title. [DNLM: 1. Epidemiology. 2. Pre-
ventive Medicine. WA 105 R515e]
RA651.R53 1987   614.4   87-17867

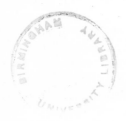

Produced by Longman Group (FE) Ltd
Printed in Hong Kong

Preface

This book is intended primarily for students of community and preventive medicine, but we hope it will also prove of value and interest to clinicians and other health professionals and to students of nursing, health visiting, health education and dentistry.

Although the study of the health of populations is at least as old as Hippocrates, it is only during the present decade that any attempt has been made to bring together the epidemiological knowledge relating to a wide spectrum of diseases. We have written this book to complement the information contained in clinical textbooks and have adopted the familiar approach of dealing with communicable diseases together (Chs 2–4) and with non-communicable diseases system by system (Chs 5–15). A brief introduction (Ch. 1) outlines the roles of epidemiology, the methods used in examining the causes of disease and the strategies used in prevention. Effective prevention of a disease usually stems from an understanding of its causes. For each disease or injury considered here, we attempt to relate the epidemiological knowledge on pathogenesis to the available preventive methods.

We have included several conditions that are usually regarded as 'tropical diseases'. This has been done to encourage a global view of medicine and to equip the reader to understand these conditions should they be imported into this country or encountered on overseas visits such as medical student electives.

We have not given a detailed bibliography but, for students wishing to enquire further into a particular topic, have included a short list of useful reference books. Where incidence and prevalence figures (numbers or rates) are given, they have been included to give the reader a feeling for the size of the problem — and with no expectation that students should memorize such data.

While writing this book we have received encouragement and advice from many colleagues. We are grateful to them all, and also to Mrs Mary Sharp and Mrs Margaret Greaves who typed the manuscript and Miss Renee Bailey who undertook the artwork.

I D G Richards

M R Baker

Contents

Contents

1

Introduction

Epidemiology is the branch of medical science concerned with studying the health of human populations. Its uses may be summarized as follows:

1. *Describing the health of populations* in terms of temporal trends and patterns of health (such as geographical and social class differences).

   Our knowledge of the health of populations is derived from routinely collected data (such as those shown in *Table 1.1*) and from specially conducted surveys.

2. *Explaining the health of populations,* based on a knowledge of the population's social and demographic features, environmental hazards, behavioural characteristics and provision of health services.

3. *Understanding diseases,* in particular their causes and natural history. Epidemiology also enables us to identify high-risk groups and provides the basis on which to introduce preventive measures.

Table 1.1 Some routinely collected health data

Mortality:	Registration of death
	Registration of stillbirth
Morbidity:	Hospital Activity Analysis
	Hospital Inpatient Enquiry
	Annual Hospital Statistical Returns
	Mental Health Enquiry
	General Household Survey
	National Cancer Registration Scheme
	Notification of infectious diseases
	Registration of congenital malformations
	Registration of the blind
	Notification of industrial diseases
	Notification of sickness absence
	Royal College of General Practitioners' National Morbidity Surveys
Demography:	Decennial population census
	Notification of birth

EPIDEMIOLOGICAL STUDIES OF AETIOLOGY

An understanding of the causes of disease often begins with an observation which may be clinical. This gives rise to a hypothesis which in turn is tested by epidemiological and genetic studies and by experiments (human or animal).

There are three kinds of epidemiological studies of aetiology: descriptive, analytic and experimental.

Descriptive studies

The distribution of the disease in different communities or in sub-groups is described in terms of:

1. The person: intrinsic factors (such as age, sex, ethnic group) and lifestyle (including a consideration of marital status, occupation, socioeconomic group and health related behaviour).
2. Place: global, national and regional variations, urban/rural differences, spatial clusters and the effects of migration.
3. Time: secular trends, seasonal fluctuations, epidemics, temporal clusters.

Many descriptive studies rely on routinely collected health data (*Table 1.1*). Sometimes the information needed to describe the disease distribution in a population is not readily available and it is necessary to conduct special surveys.

The two important limitations of descriptive studies are:

1. The available data may be defective in quality and completeness; an apparent association between a disease and a causal factor will then be spurious.
2. It is difficult to distinguish between causes of disease and factors that are fortuitously associated with the disease; for example, there may be a 'common cause' for the suspected factor and the disease.

Analytic studies

These are used to test hypotheses arising out of descriptive studies. These are of two kinds:

1. Case–control (retrospective) studies in which the diseased person's past history and exposure to suspected harmful agents are ascertained and compared with the same data collected in the same way from a control group who are individuals known to be free of the disease.
2. Cohort (prospective) studies which involve the investigation of a group of people who are identified by characteristics that are manifest before the

onset of the disease. They are followed up over a period of time and the incidence of disease is compared with the incidence in a comparison (control) group which is a cohort in whom there is no known exposure to the suspected cause.

Each type of investigation has its advantages and disadvantages. For example, case–control studies can be conducted relatively quickly and inexpensively but they rely on retrospective data which may be unreliable or incomplete. It is difficult to be sure whether a demonstrable association is causal. Cohort studies take longer and tend to be more expensive but they do permit calculation of the relative risk (the ratio of the incidence rate in the exposed group to the incidence rate in the non-exposed group) and the attributable risk (the difference between the incidence in the exposed and non-exposed groups).

Experimental studies

These provide the most convincing evidence of cause. They test whether a group of people deliberately exposed to a suspected causal agent, or protected from it, have a different incidence of disease from that of the general population. The former approach (exposure to an agent) has ethical implications and is rarely adopted except in animal experiments. Sometimes epidemiological 'experiments' are unplanned, for example nuclear explosions and accidents (followed by an increased incidence of leukaemia) and administration of high levels of oxygen to neonates (leading to retrolental fibroplasia).

THE GENESIS OF DISEASE

Many factors interact to produce disease and it is customary to divide them into three groups — the host, the agent and the environment (*Table 1.2*). The role of the environment is threefold: it influences the existence of the agent, exposure of the host to the agent, and the susceptibility of the host. The role of epidemiology is to integrate the available data on host, agent and environment and to evaluate their aetiological importance.

It is important to realize that statistical associations between the occurrence of disease and the suspected agents may be due to a third factor influencing both. Evidence of a true causal relationship includes:

1. Repeatability (consistency): the same association is found in different populations.
2. Plausibility: the association is consistent with the known activity of the suspected agent.
3. Dose–response relationship: the incidence of disease correlates with the amount and duration of exposure.

Table 1.2 Factors in the genesis of disease

The host
  Genotype
  Age
  Sex
  Ethnic group
  Physiological state: pregnancy, stress, nutrition, fatigue
  Immunological state
  Psychological state
  Pre-existing or intercurrent disease
  Behaviour: hygiene, foodhandling, exercise, diet, occupation, smoking, alcohol and drug
            abuse, sexual activity

The agent
  Infectious: bacteria, viruses, metazoa, protozoa, rickettsia, fungi
  Physical: mechanical, ionizing radiation, heat, cold
  Chemical: poisons, drugs, allergens
  Nutritional: excesses, deficiencies

The environment
  Physical: geology, climate, air, water
  Biological: human — density
            flora — food sources
            fauna — food sources, hosts and vectors of disease
  Socioeconomic: urbanization, industrialization, disruption (by wars, floods, earthquakes),
            wealth, employment

4. Experimental confirmation: the disease can be reproduced in animal experiments.
5. Temporal relationship: exposure must precede the onset of the disease.
6. Disease distribution: this should be similar to that of the supposed agent.
7. Removal: the incidence falls if the factor is removed or reduced.

THE PREVENTION OF DISEASE

Primary prevention, which is the prevention of the onset of disease, depends on effective intervention in the relationship between host, agent and environment. Strategies related to the human *host* involve:

1. Genetic counselling.
2. Health education to encourage people to behave in a way that is conducive to health.
3. Enhancement or resistance to disease by immunization or improved nutrition.
4. Chemoprophylaxis (e.g. against malaria, meningococcal meningitis or wound infection).
5. Screening to detect predisposing conditions (such as hypertension or the tuberculin negative state).

Examples of strategies related to the *agents* of disease and the *environment* are shown below.

Strategies	Examples
Destroy the agent	Chlorination of water supplies, pasteurization of milk
Reduce the 'dose' of the agent	Wet drilling in coal mines
Substitute the agent	Use of non-carcinogenic substances in industry
Inhibit transmission of the agent	Isolate cases of the infectious disease. Destroy the vectors of disease. Prevent the contamination of water, milk and food. Improve ventilation and reduce overcrowding
Prevent contact of the agent and host	Guards for machinery, protective clothing

Secondary prevention involves action to reduce the duration of disease by early detection or early diagnosis, followed by prompt, effective treatment. For some conditions, this involves screening to detect the disease in its pre-symptomatic phase.

Epidemiological studies define for us those groups in the population that are at increased risk of disease, disability, injury or death. The identification of high-risk groups enables preventive measures to be directed towards those sections of the population most likely to benefit. The term 'risk factor' denotes an attribute (such as age or ethnic group) or exposure (for example rubella in pregnancy or cigarette smoke) that is associated with an increased probability of the occurrence of disease or other specified outcome. It may indicate a causal relationship, or may merely define groups at increased risk without there being a causal link.

FURTHER READING

Epidemiological methods

Alderson M 1983 An introduction to epidemiology. 2nd edn. Macmillan Press, London

Barker D J P, Rose G 1979 Epidemiology in medical practice. 2nd edn. Churchill Livingstone, Edinburgh

Mausner J S, Kramer S 1985 Epidemiology — An introductory text. 2nd edn. Saunders, London

Rose G, Barker D J P 1986 Epidemiology for the uninitiated. 2nd edn. British Medical Association, London

Systematic epidemiology

Alderson M (ed) 1982 The prevention of cancer. Edward Arnold, London

Barron S L, Thomson A M (eds) 1983 Obstetrical epidemiology. Academic Press, London

Bourke G J (ed) 1983 The epidemiology of cancer. Croom Helm, London

Christie A B 1980 Infectious diseases: epidemiology and clinical practice. 3rd edn. Churchill Livingstone, Edinburgh

Cliff K S 1984 Accidents: Causes, prevention and services. Croom Helm, London

Freeman H (ed) 1985 Mental health and the environment. Churchill Livingstone, Edinburgh

Hunter D 1978 The diseases of occupations. 6th edn. Hodder and Stoughton, London

Kelsey J L 1982 Musculoskeletal diseases. Oxford University Press, Oxford

Langman M J S 1979 The epidemiology of chronic digestive diseases. Edward Arnold, Nottingham

McCarthy M 1982 Epidemiology and policies for health planning. King Edward's Hospital Fund for London, London

Miller D L, Farmer R D T (eds) 1979 Epidemiology of diseases. Blackwell, Oxford

Passmore R, Eastwood M A 1986 Davidson's human nutrition and dietetics. 8th edn. Churchill Livingstone, Edinburgh

Rose F C (ed) 1980 Clinical neuroepidemiology. Pitman Medical, Tunbridge Wells

Trowell H C, Burkitt D P (eds) 1981 Western diseases: their emergence and prevention. Edward Arnold, London

Vessey M P, Gray M (eds) 1985 Cancer risks and prevention. Oxford University Press, Oxford

2

Airborne infections

The spread of organisms through the air occurs in three ways:

1. Organisms are expelled from the nose or mouth of infectious persons in moist droplets which pass directly to the respiratory mucosa of a person nearby.
2. Droplets containing the organisms are carried some distance by air currents.
3. Droplets fall to the ground or other surfaces and subsequent cleaning or dusting results in a cloud of dried particles rising into the air and infecting those nearby.

Airborne infections may be classified as follows:

1. *Exanthemata* (characterized by a distinctive rash) — measles, rubella (German measles), scarlatina (scarlet fever), varicella (chicken pox).
2. *Mouth and throat infections* — diphtheria, mumps, tonsillitis.
3. *Respiratory tract infections* — pertussis (whooping cough), influenza and other virus infections, pulmonary tuberculosis.
4. *General* — infectious mononucleosis, leprosy, meningitis.

MEASLES

This acute viral infection is charaterized by fever, upper respiratory catarrh, photophobia, Koplik's spots and a generalized maculopapular rash. Complications include otitis media, pneumonia, encephalitis and bronchiectasis.

Epidemiology

Measles is transmitted through nasopharyngeal and oropharyngeal droplets expelled during coughing or sneezing by infected persons. Communicability lasts for about a week from the onset of the prodrome and is maximal just before the rash appears.

7

Measles occurs worldwide. In developing countries it is a killing disease with fatality occasionally reaching 50%. In Britain, mortality has fallen dramatically since the beginning of the century owing to the improved nutrition of the community, the use of antibiotics and, more recently, the introduction of immunization. Epidemics of measles, each lasting about 6 months, used to occur every second or third year; this is because one epidemic cannot follow another until there are sufficient non-immune children as a result of new births. Since the introduction of measles immunization on a national scale in 1968, the biennial epidemics have been much smaller. In temperate climates, outbreaks occur mainly in the late winter and early spring. In the USA, where most children are immunized, the incidence is low and epidemics no longer occur regularly.

The disease is uncommon in the first 6 months of life because of passive immunity from the mother. The highest incidence is in the age group 1–7 years. In developing countries it is common between 4 months and 2 years. It is a highly infectious desease, and the great majority of people have had an attack of measles before the end of childhood. An attack usually confers lifelong immunity.

The risk of respiratory infection is greatest in children who are socially deprived or handicapped, either physically or mentally. Neurological and respiratory complications and otitis media are still common in unvaccinated children. The younger the patient, the greater the risk of death. It has been widely assumed that malnutrition predisposes to severe infection but recent evidence suggests that prolonged and intense exposure from infected siblings is a more important determinant.

Prevention

Because maternal antibodies can persist for up to 12 months, measles immunization is usually delayed in the UK until the second year of life. A single injection of live attenuated virus should be given early in the second year but there is no upper age limit. The World Health Organization recommends immunizing at 9 months and that is probably appropriate for developing countries because the disease tends to occur at a younger age. It is particularly important that the following high-risk groups are immunized:

1. Children from the age of 1 year upwards who are in special care.
2. Children entering nursery school or other establishment accepting children for day care.
3. Children with serious physical incapacity who are likely to develop serious illness as a result of natural measles infection.

Mass immunization is also important in areas such as West Africa where measles is a serious infection carrying high fatality. The vaccine is contraindicated in children with malignant disease, hypogammaglobulinaemia, an acute illness or allergy to hen's egg. Corticosteroid and immunosuppressive therapy are also contraindications. Susceptible debilitated child contacts can be protected with human normal immunoglobulin but the protection lasts for only 3–6 weeks.

An immunization level of at least 80% is required to control the disease; our failure to do this in Britain has been due to low acceptance rates (50–60%). In developing countries preventive measures will also include better nutrition, breast feeding, wider spacing of children and provision of adequate housing. Isolation does little to prevent infection in family contacts, and quarantine of school contacts is unnecessary.

Measles is a notifiable disease in the UK. These notifications provide information on long-term trends in the disease and facilitate the early detection of epidemics.

RUBELLA (GERMAN MEASLES)

Rubella is a mild infectious disease characterized by a discrete macular rash, enlargement of the posterior cervical lymph nodes and occasionally an arthritis. Its importance lies in its teratogenic effects.

Epidemiology

Rubella is spread by respiratory droplets, except for intra-uterine infection which occurs by the transplacental route. The disease occurs throughout the world; cases occur sporadically with occasional local epidemics. Before the introduction of vaccine, epidemics occurred at approximately 7 year intervals. In the UK, the disease usually reaches a peak in June or July each year. Rubella is most common in schoolchildren and young adults; by adult life 85% show serological evidence of previous infection although many have no history of a rash and may be unaware of having had the infection.

Infection is spread by droplet spray from the nasopharyngeal secretions during the acute phase of the disease which is from about 5 days before the rash appears to about 5 days after it has faded. Rubella was thought to convey permanent immunity but second attacks undoubtedly occur.

Rubella in the first 4 months of pregnancy may give rise to congenital abnormalities which are collectively referred to as the 'rubella syndrome'. Most common are deafness, cardiac malformation (patent ductus arteriosus and septal defects) and cataracts. Microcephaly, mental retardation, hepatosplenomegaly and thrombocytopenic purpura may also occur. Spontaneous abortion and stillbirth rates are raised following rubella in the first trimester. Babies infected *in utero* can excrete the virus for months after birth. Fetal damage is highest (more than 50%) if the infection is contracted in the first 4 weeks after conception; average figures for the second and third months are 25% and 10% respectively.

Prevention

Isolation of cases and quarantine of contacts are unnecessary. Pregnant women should avoid exposure to the infection. If a woman in early pregnancy is a close contact of rubella, her serum should be examined. If it contains rubella antibody and the incubation period has not passed, she will not contract the disease. It may be worthwhile giving immunoglobulin if no antibody is present, but studies by the Public Health Laboratory Service have shown that it cannot be relied upon to prevent infection, either clinical or subclinical.

The policy in the UK is to increase the proportion of women who are fully protected by immunizing (using a live attenuated vaccine) girls between their 10th and 14th birthdays irrespective of a history of rubella (which cannot be relied on as evidence of actual immunity since rashes that look like rubella may occur during other infections).

Immunization is also strongly recommended for:

1. Seronegative women with an occupational risk of acquiring rubella, e.g. nurses, teachers and virus laboratory staff.
2. Women found by routine screening during pregnancy to be seronegative; for them, immunization is advised in the postpartum period.

Precautions should be taken against becoming pregnant for 3 months after immunization in order to avoid the possible risk of harm to the fetus. Termination of pregnancy is usually recommended in the event of inadvertent vaccination during the first 2 months even though the vaccine strain appears to be far less teratogenic.

SCARLATINA (SCARLET FEVER)

Scarlet fever is caused by *Streptococcus pyogenes* of Lancefield's Group A. Streptococcal tonsillitis is the same disease but without the effects of erythrogenic toxin. A large proportion of the population harbours the organism in the throat.

Epidemiology

Scarlatina is found in the world's temperate zones. Over recent centuries the disease has waxed and waned in severity several times for no obvious reason and at present it is a mild condition. The maximum incidence is in the age group 5–10 years.

Transmission is normally from a case or carrier by droplet infection. However, explosive outbreaks have occurred as a result of infected milk and ice-cream. Infected dust and articles (such as crockery and pencils) may transmit the infection. Hospital infection with haemolytic streptococcus is an important problem; carriers (among staff or patients), infected wounds, burns and umbilical stumps act as sources of cross-infection.

Prevention

The patient is isolated at home until the fever and symptoms have subsided. Removal to hospital may occasionally be required, e.g. if there is gross over-crowding, or a recently delivered mother in the household, or if a member of the family works in a dairy. If the patient or a close contact is returning to a residential school or to an occupation which carries a particular risk (food or milk handling, nursing, midwifery), nose and throat swabs should be negative.

Institutional outbreaks as in hospitals or schools are managed by daily clinical inspection and routine nose, throat and wounds swabbing and exclusion of those found to be carrying the organism until treatment has produced a bacteriological cure. Medical and nursing staff should report sore throats and be managed as above. Prophylactic oral penicillin has been successful in controlling institutional outbreaks of streptococcal infection.

VARICELLA (CHICKENPOX)

Chickenpox is a mild, highly infectious disease caused by the varicella-zoster virus. The virus may be isolated from the nasopharynx of cases and from fresh vesicular skin lesions. Infectivity lasts from the onset of symptoms until the skin lesions become crusted.

Epidemiology

It occurs throughout the world and is endemic in all large cities. Local epidemics occur at irregular intervals. The disease, which occurs mainly in childhood, confers permanent immunity. Transmission is usually by droplet infection, either from the respiratory tract (for several days before the rash appears) or from vesicle fluid (in the first 3 or 4 days of the lesions). Following primary infection, the virus remains dormant in dorsal root ganglia.

Patients with herpes zoster (shingles) can transmit chickenpox, but herpes zoster cannot be contracted from a patient with chickenpox. Herpes zoster is caused by reactivation of the virus which has remained dormant in the dorsal root ganglion after a previous attack of chickenpox. It is a sporadic disease which occurs with increasing frequency with age.

Prevention

Cases of chickenpox are kept indoors until the lesions have crusted. Human immunoglobulin is available for susceptible contacts with immunodeficiency, such as children having immunosuppressive treatment. There is no way of preventing herpes zoster infection.

DIPHTHERIA

Diphtheria is caused by *Corynebacterium diphtheriae* and is characterized by membrane formation in the throat and the absorption of an endotoxin which damages heart muscle and nervous tissue. The fatality rate is 5–10%, death being due usually to asphyxia or heart failure.

Epidemiology

In many parts of the world, diphtheria is common and fatality is high. Earlier this century there were 50 000 cases and 4000 deaths each year in Britain alone. In most developed countries, immunization has resulted in the virtual disappearance of the disease; in Britain, the introduction of intensive community immunization in 1940 resulted in a rapid decline in the incidence (*Fig. 2.1*). When cases occur, they are mainly due to the *mitis* strain, in contrast to the preponderance of infections by the *gravis* strain in the pre-immunization era. Transmission is principally by droplet infection from a case or carrier, although indirect spread (via infected articles) and milk-borne epidemics can occur. Wound diphtheria sometimes occurs, especially during hostilities in poor countries.

Prevention

The disease can be prevented by active immunization. Diphtheria toxoid (as a component of triple vaccine) is available for immunization in the first year of life; a booster dose (combined with tetanus toxoid) is given at school entry. Adults requiring protection are Schick tested first and positive reactors receive active immunization. Alternatively, they may be given a low-dose adsorbed diphtheria toxoid vaccine without being Schick tested.

Suspected cases are admitted immediately to an isolation hospital pending confirmation of the diagnosis. Cases and carriers are sought among school contacts and households by throat inspection and by nasal and throat swabbing. Immunized contacts are given a booster dose of diphtheria toxoid; non-immunized contacts are given a small dose of antitoxin and active immunization is commenced.

Importation of the disease can be expected from time to time and spread

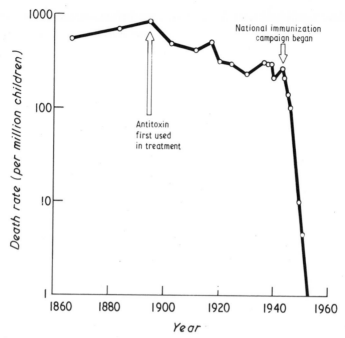

Fig. 2.1 Diphtheria: death rates for children under 15 in England and Wales.

among the unimmunized members of the community may occur. However, it will not become re-established in this country if infant immunization rates of 80–90% are maintained.

MUMPS

Mumps (infectious parotitis) is a viral disease characterized by enlargement of the parotid and/or other salivary glands. Subclinical infections are common. Complications are common, especially orchitis (which occurs in about 20% of post-pubertal male cases) and viral meningitis. Sterility following orchitis is rare. Deafness as a complication of mumps is also rare.

Epidemiology

Mumps occurs throughout the world and is endemic in Britain. Epidemics occur approximately every 7 years but localized outbreaks occur from time to time, especially in residential institutions. The source of infection is the saliva of a case and transmission is by droplet infection, oral contact or recently contaminated articles. It is mainly a disease of children and adolescents; sub-clinical infections are common and most people will have had the disease by middle age. Infectivity lasts from a few days before salivary gland swelling begins until the glands have completely regressed. Immunity is usually permanent.

Prevention

Isolation of cases and quarantine of contacts are unnecessary. A live attenuated vaccine can be given to adults and children over 1 year of age. It may also be used for susceptible post-pubertal males who wish to avoid the possibility of developing mumps but routine immunization is not considered justified in the UK.

PERTUSSIS (WHOOPING COUGH)

Whooping cough is a respiratory illness caused by the organism *Bordetella pertussis*. It is characterized by paroxysmal coughing, often accompanied by the typical respiratory 'whoop'. Numerous inapparent and atypical cases occur, and the characteristic features of the illness can also be caused by *B. parapertussis* and some adenoviruses.

Epidemiology

Whooping cough occurs throughout the world. The incidence depends largely on the level of local immunity; it affects mainly children under the age of 7 years. The severity depends on age, with the majority of complicated cases and deaths occurring in infants, particularly in those under 6 months of age. Deaths from pertussis have not been reported in fully immunized infants. In developing countries, and before immunization became available, fatality could exceed 10%.

Transmission is mainly by droplet infection. It is a highly infectious disease, and few susceptible home contacts escape. One attack usually produces substantial immunity but second attacks have been reported. An infant is susceptible from birth, there being no passive immunity from the mother.

The incidence of whooping cough in Britain began to fall when immunization was introduced on a national scale in 1957 although mortality had been falling since the end of the last century (*Fig. 2.2*). In the decade prior to 1957, the average annual number of notifications was over 100 000; in the following two decades it was under 30 000 and under 10 000 respectively. Adverse publicity about pertussis immunization has resulted in a reduction in the level of immunity and a consequent increase in the incidence of the disease; this is generally accepted as evidence of the effectiveness of the vaccine in the prevention of clinical cases. The case fatality rate fell from over 10 deaths per 1000 cases notified in the early 1940s to about one death per 1000 cases in

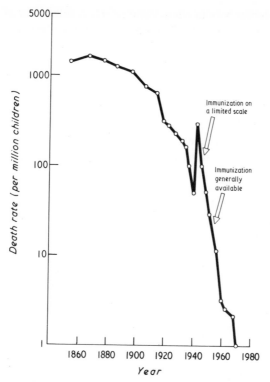

Fig. 2.2 Whooping cough: death rates for children under 15 in England and Wales.

1953–56. It remained unchanged for the next 20 years but dropped abruptly to about 0.2 per 1000 cases after 1976.

Prevention

The patient must be isolated until considered non-infectious; infectivity begins with the onset of catarrhal symptoms and lasts for up to a month, but not usually as long as the cough. Infants who accidentally come into contact with the disease should receive prophylactic erythromycin and be protected from further exposure. Quarantine of school contacts is unnecessary.

Immunization against pertussis is effective in keeping the herd immunity high enough to prevent outbreaks, provided the uptake is at least 70%. When the uptake has fallen to 30–40% as a result of adverse publicity about vaccine safety, epidemics have occurred. Active immunization with killed organisms is given to 3-month-old infants and repeated after 6–8 weeks and again after 6 months. The reason that the first dose is delayed until 3 months is that, at earlier ages, the immune response is poor.

Pertussis vaccines vary in efficacy and safety. A full course of vaccine confers protection in over 80% of the recipients, and the severity of the illness is less in those who do contract the disease despite immunization. A very small proportion of immunized children have experienced neurological complications such as convulsions and persistent screaming. Permanent brain damage to young children from whooping cough vaccine appears to be a rare event (estimated at about 1 in 310 000 injections) and the benefits conferred by immunization are considered to outweigh the very small risk of serious neurological reactions that may arise.

The contraindications to pertussis immunization accepted in Britain are as follows:

1. Any acute febrile illness, particularly respiratory, until fully recovered. Minor infections without fever or systemic upset are not regarded as a contraindication.
2. A history of any severe local or general reaction (including a neurological reaction) to a preceding dose; or a history of cerebral irritation or damage in the neonatal period; or a history of fits or convulsions.

There are certain groups of children in whom whooping cough immunization is not absolutely contraindicated but who require special consideration as to its advisability. These groups are: children whose parents or siblings have a history of idiopathic epilepsy, children with developmental delay thought to be due to a neurological defect and children with neurological disease. For these groups the risk of immunization may be higher than in normal children but the effects of whooping cough may be more severe, so that the benefits of immunization would also be greater. The balance of risk and benefit should be assessed with special care in each individual case.

A personal or family history of allergy has in the past been regarded as a contraindication to immunization but there is now a substantial body of medical opinion which no longer considers this to be so. Doctors should, however, use their own discretion in the individual case. Even when pertussis vaccine is contraindicated, an infant should still be considered for immunization against diphtheria and tetanus.

INFLUENZA AND OTHER ACUTE RESPIRATORY INFECTIONS

A wide range of microorganisms, especially viruses and bacteria, cause respiratory infections. Viruses may produce characteristic syndromes and, at other times, simple upper respiratory tract infections. Bacteria are usually secondary invaders in a viral infection or in an already damaged lung.

Epidemiology

It is the very young child and the chronic bronchitic that suffer the most serious infections. Globally, acute respiratory infections are one of the major causes of mortality. Influenza A is responsible for widespread epidemics or pandemics of influenza; the virus has the capacity to develop new antigenic variants at irregular intervals. In recent decades, pandemics occurred in 1957 ('Asian influenza'), 1967 ('Hong Kong influenza') and 1972. Influenza B is associated with localized outbreaks and sporadic cases, usually of a milder nature, about every second year.

The highest incidence of influenza occurs in the winter months. Infectivity is high and extends from shortly before symptoms occur until shortly after the pyrexia settles. Transmission is generally by droplet infection.

In patients with the common cold, it has proved impossible to isolate a virus in more than half the cases; rhinoviruses and coronavirus are those most consistently isolated. Transmission from the upper respiratory tract of cases is by droplet infection or close personal contact; it is facilitated by overcrowding and poor ventilation. Infectivity is high in the early stages. The incidence falls with age, presumably due to an increasing level of immunity. Lowered resistance due to fatigue or other causes may predispose to an attack.

Postoperative pneumonia has not changed appreciably in incidence over the past 30 years. Surveys have shown an incidence around 20% following upper abdominal surgery; it is negligible after surgery outside the chest and abdomen in fit patients. The risk is increased in smokers and patients with chronic respiratory disease or obesity.

Prevention

Immunization plays a limited role in the control of influenza. A new vaccine has to be prepared each time the virus changes and at the time of an epidemic it tends to be in short supply. Afterwards, immunization is recommended only for special groups such as patients with chronic lung or heart disease and key hospital staff. No effective vaccine is yet available for the prevention of the common cold.

PULMONARY TUBERCULOSIS

This is a chronic infection produced by the human strain of *Mycobacterium tuberculosis*. Infection with tubercule bacilli does not usually result in disease but, in a minority, the initial exposure will result in primary tuberculosis consisting of a small subpleural lesion and enlarged hilar and mediastinal glands. Postprimary tuberculosis varies enormously in its extent and speed of progression — from an indolent form with a well-circumscribed cavity to a rapidly progressing disease with caseation, irregular cavitation and extensive bronchopneumonia.

Epidemiology

Pulmonary tuberculosis remains one of the most important communicable diseases in the world today, with an estimated 50 million active cases and an annual mortality of 3 million. In tropical countries such as India and Pakistan, 1–2% of the population have active pulmonary tuberculosis. In Britain, there has been a rapid decline in mortality and morbidity rates during this century, the decline being greatest in young adults among whom notification rates were at one time highest.

This trend (due largely to improved nutrition of the community and a reduction in domestic overcrowding) began long before the introduction of specific preventive measures, although the rate of fall accelerated after effective chemotherapy and specific preventive measures became available (*Fig. 2.3*). Postprimary tuberculosis now occurs most often in middle-aged and elderly men and in Asian immigrants. About 10 000 new cases of pulmonary tuberculosis are notified each year in England and Wales, of which about a quarter are sputum positive (i.e. acid-fast bacilli are seen on a smear).

Transmission takes place by droplet infection or by close personal contact. During a primary infection, sensitivity to tuberculo-protein develops and the

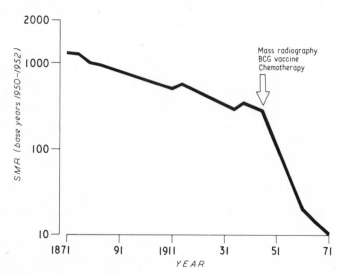

Fig. 2.3 Tuberculosis: mortality in 1871–1971 in England and Wales. (SMR = Standardized mortality ratio.)

tuberculin skin test becomes positive about 6 weeks after the onset of the infection. At the age of 13 years, about 8% of British schoolchildren have a positive tuberculin test, although the milder reactions are non-specific.

Prevention

The most important preventive measure is treatment of sputum-positive individuals. Infectious cases of pulmonary tuberculosis are treated in hospital until the sputum culture is negative. Bacteriological cure is now possible in over 90% of cases. Protracted treatment is needed to achieve sterilization of the lesion and patient compliance may be a problem. In developing countries, the cost of drugs reduces the contribution of chemotherapy in the control of tuberculosis.

A search is made for cases among patients' contacts at school, at work and in the home; adults are X-rayed and children receive a tuberculin test. Positive reactors have an X-ray; tuberculin negative contacts are vaccinated.

· Bacille Calmette-Guérin (BCG) vaccine is made from a live attenuated strain of bovine tuberculosis and is given intracutaneously. In Britain it is offered to children between their 10th and 14th birthdays and to contacts of known cases; a preliminary tuberculin test is performed to eliminate positive reactors for whom the vaccine is contraindicated.

Since there is no transfer of immunity to a baby from its mother, BCG vaccine should be offered at birth for infants born into households where there is active tuberculosis. It should also be considered for immigrants from developing countries. Although results in some countries have not been impressive, in Britain BCG immunization at adolescence resulted in a 75% reduction in the incidence of tuberculosis in the succeeding 10 years.

Mass miniature radiography of apparently healthy individuals has now been discontinued in Britain because of the low yield — generally less than 1 active case per 1000 examined. The examination of certain high incidence groups, such as immigrants, mental hosptial patients and casual lodging house users, continues to be worthwhile.

INFECTIOUS MONONUCLEOSIS (GLANDULAR FEVER)

This is a benign febrile illness characterized by lymphadenopathy, atypical monocytes in the peripheral blood and a positive Paul–Bunnell reaction. It is caused by the Epstein–Barr virus.

Epidemiology

The disease occurs in most parts of the world but its incidence is difficult to estimate in Britain because it is not generally notifiable. Cases are usually sporadic and mainly in young adults, but prolonged localized epidemics sometimes occur, usually in schools and institutions. The virus is excreted in the oropharyngeal secretions during the illness and for some months afterwards. Spread is probably by droplet infection although kissing has also been incriminated.

Infectivity is not high but surveys show that mild or subclinical infections are very common from an early age. Mortality is very low; most reported deaths follow a neurological complication.

Prevention

Infectious mononucleosis is not highly contagious and neither isolation of cases nor quarantine of contacts is necessary.

LEPROSY

Leprosy is a chronic disease caused by *Mycobacterium leprae*. It has a long incubation period of about 3 years. The infection may be a transient skin patch (indeterminate leprosy) or a more chronic well-defined patch or patches (tuberculoid leprosy). Poor resistance to leprosy may lead to it becoming a generalized infection of the skin, nasal mucosa and even of organs like the liver (lepromatous leprosy). Nerve damage may occur in any of these kinds of leprosy.

Epidemiology

Leprosy is important because it cripples; if 'crippling' is taken to include impairment of sensation, then about a quarter of those suffering from leprosy are crippled. It is thus the cause of grave economic loss in many developing countries. It is also a disease that has serious social consequence for the patient and his family. Probably only one in every five cases is at present able to obtain treatment.

The prevalence of leprosy is unknown and the often quoted world total of 15 million is likely to be an underestimate. The total prevalence is probably increasing, and this for several reasons. In very few countries have leprosy control schemes been successfully organized, medical facilities are often inadequate in the rural parts of countries with a large leprosy problem, populations in those countries are increasing and the life span is lengthening. Because of fear or the shame felt by many leprosy patients, the disease may be hidden by the patients and their families. This leads to under-reporting of cases and in turn to incomplete statistics about the distribution of the disease.

Most cases are found in the populous countries of South-East Asia and in

Africa and South America; it is estimated that there are almost four million cases in India alone. In such countries, a high prevalence of leprosy is to be found in patients attending skin and orthopaedic clinics and in beggars. In the UK, approximately 20 new cases are diagnosed annually and there are about 350 registered active cases; all of these have acquired the infection abroad.

Leprosy is largely an airborne infection, the organism being spread by the watery discharge from the nose, although some spread takes place by direct close contact. Resistance to infection varies considerably; a small proportion of the population is very susceptible and will succumb to the severe type of disease if exposed. Patients with early leprosy are not ill and suffer from no deformities. Lactating women with untreated lepromatous leprosy discharge enormous numbers of *M.leprae* in their milk.

Prevention

The control of leprosy, which is a mildly contagious disease, can include some or all of the following measures:

1. *Segregation of infectious cases.* This is quite impossible in any developing country; it is too costly, leads to concealment of cases and is likely to result in the segregation of those with obvious deformities rather than patients suffering from infectious kinds of the disease.
2. *Raising the general standard of living and hygiene and the abolition of domestic overcrowding.* This may explain the decline of leprosy in the north-west of Europe and point the way to control elsewhere. In most countries where leprosy is a serious problem, this is impossible.
3. *Prophylaxis.* The twice weekly oral administration of dapsone to healthy individuals for several years is generally impracticable and, because it is potentially a toxic drug, it may be undesirable.
4. *B C G vaccination.* This method of leprosy control is still the subject of investigation.
5. *Reduction of the reservoir of infection.* This is at present the most certain measure that can generally be adopted. There is no intermediate host of *M.leprae* and, as far as is known, the organism is found only in man. Reducing the human reservoir of infection by means of treatment of the patient suffering from active leprosy would appear to hold out the greatest chances of success in controlling the disease. Since the number of people presenting at a clinic for diagnosis and treatment bears no relationship to the size of the leprosy endemic, it is important that annual whole-population surveys should be conducted. Where the prevalence of leprosy exceeds 1% in a community, everybody must be considered to be a potential contact. In addition there should be surveys of people at special risk,

such as household and family contacts of known leprosy cases. Quarterly or 6-monthly examination of such contacts is recommended.

MENINGITIS

The organisms which commonly cause acute meningitis are: *Neisseria meningitidis*, *Streptococcus pneumoniae*, *Haemophilus influenzae* and the Echo and Coxsackie groups of viruses. Some of these infections are still associated with a high fatality, much of which is related to delay in making a correct diagnosis.

Epidemiology

Meningococcal meningitis (due to *Neisseria meningitidis*) is mainly a disease of children. It is the commonest cause of bacterial meningitis in UK. The organism is often found in the nasopharynx of asymptomatic carriers. Spread is by droplets and infection occurs most frequently in the winter and spring. It may reach epidemic proportions in overcrowded conditions.

Pneumococcal meningitis (due to *Streptococcus pneumoniae*) usually occurs as a result of septicaemic spread of infection from a focus in the lungs, sinuses or middle ear. Young infants and adults over 40 are most commonly involved. In people over 50, the fatality rate may be as high as 50%.

Haemophilus influenzae meningitis is almost exclusively a disease of infants and children of pre-school age. The mortality from this form of meningitis is still 5–10% and some survivors may be left with a degree of mental retardation. Epidemiological studies have shown an incresed risk of spread within the families of cases.

Viruses are probably responsible for about 80% of all cases of meningitis in Britain, although a positive culture is obtained in only a small proportion. In some parts of the world, poliomyelitis is still an important cause of aseptic meningitis.

Prevention

Little can be done to prevent sporadic outbreaks of meningococcal infection. Provided the organism is sensitive, a short course of sulphonamide will destroy the organisms in carriers and among family and school contacts. Epidemics may be terminated by adequate bed spacing and ventilation in institutions, and the prophylactic use of sulphonamides.

3

Infections acquired by mouth

Diseases resulting from the ingestion of pathogenic organisms are common throughout the world; in developing countries they remain a leading cause of death, especially among young children. Such diseases are acquired from both human and animal sources. Examples are:

Human sources	*Animal sources*
Amoebiasis	Bacterial food poisoning
Bacillary dysentery	Bovine tuberculosis
Cholera	Brucellosis
Enteric fever	Hydatid disease
Gastroenteritis	Roundworm and tapeworm infections
Hepatitis A (infectious hepatitis)	
Poliomyelitis	

Transmission from human sources, whether cases or carriers, may be either (1) direct via contaminated hands, clothing, etc.; or (2) indirect via food or water.

Most of these infections are acquired exclusively by the oral route but some, such as hepatitis A and poliomyelitis, may be transmitted by other routes as well.

AMOEBIASIS

Entamoeba hystolytica is a protozoon with a cystic and a trophozoite stage. Ingested cysts release trophozoites which invade the gut wall, causing amoebic dysentery, or pass to the liver via the portal circulation.

Epidemiology

Amoebiasis is found in countries where standards of hygiene and sanitation are poor. It is common in tropical and subtropical regions; in such areas, more than 10% of the population may have a chronic *E. histolytica* infection of the large intestine. It occurs mainly in adults; amoebic dysentery and liver abscess are both more common in men.

Man is the main reservoir of infection. Cysts are passed in the stools of asymptomatic carriers; infection is usually from food contaminated by faecally soiled fingers or by the use of human faeces as fertilizer.

Prevention

Asymptomatic patients who are passing the cysts in the stool should have the infection eradicated by drug therapy, but prevention depends principally on personal hygiene, effective sanitary arrangements and either the avoidance of human faeces as a fertilizer or their composting before use.

BACILLARY DYSENTERY (SHIGELLOSIS)

This is an acute, usually mild, disease characterized by diarrhoea with blood and mucus in the stools and caused by *Shigella* of which there are four subgroups: *Sh. dysenteriae*, *Sh. flexneri*, *Sh. boydii* and *Sh. sonnei*.

Epidemiology

The disease is common throughout the world and remains endemic even in developed countries. The incidence is highest in tropical countries, where dysentery occurs in both endemic and epidemic forms. Dysentery in developed countries is principally due to *Sh. sonnei*; elsewhere *Sh. flexneri* is mainly responsible.

Acute cases of dysentery are far more infectious than symptomless carriers. Infection is usually by person-to-person spread and occurs most often in overcrowded families, in institutions with poor hygienic standards and whenever sanitary arrangements are inadequate such as on the battlefield. Water-borne outbreaks (which are apt to be explosive) are uncommon, as are food-borne outbreaks in countries with high standards of hygiene. Sonné dysentery is highly infectious, and in Britain it is largely a disease of children. School outbreaks are usually due to hand-to-hand spread from the water closet.

Prevention

The basis of prevention is the disposal of human faeces in such a way that contact with hands, food or water cannot occur. In Britian, prevention is particularly dependent on toilet hygiene in nurseries and infant schools; acute cases should be excluded from school. Infected food handlers should be excluded from work until three stool cultures are negative.

CHOLERA

Caused by *Vibrio cholerae*, the typical case is characterized by copious fluid ('rice water') stools. The fluid loss often leads to severe dehydration and shock, but prompt and efficient treatment will reduce case fatality rates to a low level. Mild or asymptomatic cases are frequent and a persistent carrier state is common.

Epidemiology

The disease is endemic in the Ganges Delta and periodically spreads outwards to cause worldwide epidemics. Before 1960 these were caused by the classic biotype of *V. cholerae*. The current pandemic, which began in 1961, is due to the El Tor biotype (El Tor is a quarantine station in West Sinai); it began in Indonesia and spread throughout South East and South Asia, the Middle East and portions of Europe.

Man is the only known source. Large numbers of the organism are excreted in the diarrhoeal stools, but asymptomatic cases are also infectious and spread the disease. The commonest vehicle is water; cholera does not spread readily from person to person. In much of the developing world, contamination of water by human faeces is a frequent occurrence. When this happens, *V. cholerae* can be isolated from polluted river or well water. The organism has sometimes found its way into a normally safe public water supply with catastrophic results. Seafoods can become contaminated and will spread the disease if eaten raw or semi-cooked; other foods become contaminated if they are washed in infected water.

Cholera is a disease of poor environmental conditions and is related to overcrowding and lack of sanitation. The movement of populations, as in pilgrimages, is a potent factor in its spread.

In endemic areas, the disease attacks more children than adults, presumably because of acquired immunity in adults. When the disease moves to non-endemic areas, adults are more often affected, presumably because of the degree of exposure.

Prevention

In 1854, John Snow (anaesthetist to Queen Victoria and general practitioner) suspected that the concentration of cholera cases in the Soho district of London was the result of drinking the water from the Broad Street pump. Removal of the pump handle brought the epidemic to an end, although the microbial cause of cholera was not discovered until many years later.

The key to control lies in effective sewage disposal, care in the preparation and handling of food, and sterilization of water for drinking and food preparation. Cholera vaccine gives only partial protection and for up to 6 months only. The international spread of cholera cannot be prevented by either immunization or chemoprophylaxis, but the former is probably advisable before travelling in tropical or semi-tropical areas.

ENTERIC FEVER

'Enteric fever' is a term that embraces two diseases — typhoid fever (due to *Salmonella typhi*) and paratyphoid fever (due to *Salmonella paratyphi*). Paratyphoid fever is a milder illness with a shorter incubation period. Convalescent carriage of the organism is common but it usually clears spontaneously. *S. typhi* infection of the gall-bladder persists in about 3% of cases.

Epidemiology

Enteric fever is endemic in Africa, Central and South America, the Middle and Far East, and Southern and Eastern Europe. It is uncommon in the Western world, and the majority of cases in Britain are acquired abroad.

S. typhi is exclusively a human pathogen; *S. paratyphi* is essentially a human pathogen but infection occasionally occurs in cattle. Transmission is through the faeces or urine of a patient or carrier. The organisms can survive for long periods in water and sewage. Water-borne outbreaks of typhoid fever tend to be explosive, e.g. the outbreak in Croydon in 1937 which was due to a typhoid carrier working in a well from which the town drew its water supply. Shellfish (which filter the water in which they live), milk and cream have been responsible for spreading enteric fever. Infection can also be spread by meat and equipment used in food processing, although food-borne infection is much less common than other methods of transmission. An outbreak of over 500 cases in Aberdeen in 1964 was due to canned meat that had become contaminated by cooling the cans in sewage-polluted river water, the organisms entering the cans through minute leaks in the seal.

Prevention

This depends on the isolation and treatment of cases, detection and surveillance of carriers, provision of a pure water supply, an effective sewage system, milk pasteurization and hygienic standards in the preparation and distribution of food. Killed vaccines give partial protection (probably around 70%) for up to 5 years, and immunization is recommended for visitors to endemic areas. Carriers of the diseases should be excluded from certain occupations, such as food-handling.

GASTROENTERITIS

This is the syndrome of diarrhoea and/or vomiting which is of acute onset and of infective origin. In infants and young children, most cases are of viral origin, the rotavirus being the most important. *Escherichia coli* is the most commonly recognized bacterial cause in Britain. *Campylobacter* is also a significant cause of human diarrhoea. Bacteriological investigations of traveller's diarrhoea are often negative.

Epidemiology

It is estimated that 500 million episodes of diarrhoea occur each year among infants and young children in Asia, Africa and Latin America. Millions of babies die of gastroenteritis each year in developing countries. In developed countries, the disease is still among the leading causes of hospital admission in children under 5. It has been estimated that 5% of infants in the UK develop acute gastroenteritis, of whom 10% require admission to hospital. Poverty and poor sanitation are major contributory factors.

Rotaviruses cause gastroenteritis in infants and young children in many parts of the world; infections are more common in cold and wet seasons. *E. coli* gastroenteritis occurs most often in infants and it has been shown that infection, as opposed to illness, is very common. Spread of *E. coli* and rotaviruses occcurs rapidly in nurseries and children's wards. They are excreted in faeces and contamination of hands leads to the organisms being spread to other babies.

Campylobacter infection is most common in older children and adults. Person-to-person spread is uncommon, the majority of cases being by direct transmission from animals such as cows, dogs, sheep, cats and chickens.

Gastroenteritis due to *Giardia lamblia* is usually due to faecal–oral spread in children and probably the result of water-borne transmission in the adult.

Parvovirus-like agents are causes of the syndrome of winter vomiting disease. Transmission is considered to be by the faecal–oral route.

Prevention

Breast feeding affords protection because the milk cannot become contaminated and because it contains immunoglobulins, lactoferrin and a high concentration of lactose. The feeds for bottle-fed infants must be prepared with aseptic precautions. In hospital, an infant with gastroenteritis should be isolated from other infants and scrupulous care taken to avoid carrying the organisms to other babies.

HEPATITIS A (INFECTIOUS HEPATITIS)

Viral hepatitis is acquired by ingestion (hepatitis A) or by blood transfusion or injection (hepatitis B and non-A/non-B hepatitis).

Epidemiology

Hepatitis A virus exists worldwide and there are frequent reports of epidemics. It is spread mainly by the faecal–oral route. The prevalence of antibodies increases with age, in one study up to 92% over the age of 50 years. In temperate climates the peak incidence of symptoms occurs in winter or early spring. Poor socioeconomic conditions are associated with high infection rates. Prolonged contact is an important factor in the spread, e.g. in nurseries and residential schools. There have also been many reports of food-borne and water-borne outbreaks. There is no known carrier state and no evidence of progression to liver damage — although occasional deaths occur, probably due to liver failure.

Prevention

Once jaundice occurs, the patient is probably no longer infectious. General preventive measures include care by nurses in handling urine and faeces, good sanitation in institutions and high standards of hygiene among food-handlers.

POLIOMYELITIS

Poliomyelitis presents as a viral meningitis, complicated in severe cases by paralysis resulting from infection of the grey matter of the anterior horn of the spinal cord. The disease is caused by poliovirus which exists in three antigenically distinct types (1, 2 and 3) of which Type 1 is the most virulent. Most infections are asymptomatic and provide lifelong immunity.

Epidemiology

Before 1947, the disease was uncommon in Britain; paralytic cases were mainly very young children, hence the name 'infantile paralysis'. The virus was probably widespread in the community and subclinical infection led to immunity at a young age. In 1947 a series of yearly epidemics began, mainly due to the Type 1 virus; epidemics also occurred in other developed coun-

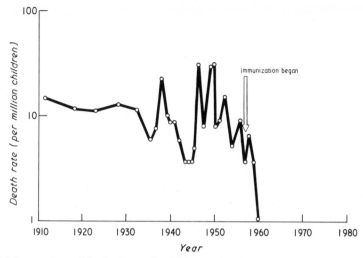

Fig. 3.1 Acute poliomyelitis: death rates for children aged under 15 years in England and Wales.

tries. This change is probably due to the rise in hygienic standards leading to large numbers of children escaping infection and the consequent development of immunity. One-third of the paralytic cases were over the age of 15 years.

The introduction of poliomyelitis immunization in 1956, at first with killed virus (Salk) vaccine and later with live attenuated virus (Sabin) vaccine, led to the virtual elimination of the disease from Britain (*Fig. 3.1*). It remains common in countries outside north-west Europe and North America. In countries with little or no immunization, the pattern resembles that seen in the pre-vaccine era in poor socioeconomic conditions: immunization of 80–90% of the population by the wild virus and sporadic cases in young children. In developing countries with partial immunization, the combination of a build-up of susceptible people, poor socioeconomic conditions and inadequate water supply systems lead to large-scale epidemics when virulent strains of the virus are introduced, often from outside the area.

The disease is spread principally by the faecal–oral route but sometimes by droplet infection. Case-fatality is around 10%, being highest in young adults. Paralysis tends to be more severe in adult cases.

Prevention

Importation of the disease into Britain, and other countries where it has been controlled, must be expected occasionally. Unimmunized people may develop poliomyelitis but the disease will not become re-established if immunization acceptance rates are in excess of 70%.

Killed vaccine cannot give rise to vaccine-associated poliomyelitis, but it has to be given by injection and it is expensive to produce. In contrast, live attenuated virus is given by mouth, it colonizes the gut promoting intestinal immunity and serum antibody production, and is cheaper to produce. Its disadvantage is that the virus is excreted in the faeces and it can cause vaccine virus infection with paralysis in close contacts. Immunization with oral vaccine should begin at 3 months of age, with the second and third doses being given at intervals of 6–8 weeks and 4–6 months respectively. Unimmunized parents of a child being given oral polio vaccine should also be offered a course; if the mother is pregnant, immunization should be delayed until after the fourth month, unless there is a risk of infection from an outbreak.

Patients in the acute stage of the disease should be barrier nursed. Pharyngeal secretions and faeces of cases and contacts are potentially dangerous and should be treated with antiseptic and disposed of as soon and as safely as possible. Contacts of cases are given oral poliomyelitis vaccine and kept under observation for 3 weeks from the last known contact.

During epidemics, children should avoid crowds; tonsillectomy and dental extractions should be postponed since they increase the risk of bulbar poliomyelitis.

BACTERIAL FOOD POISONING

The term 'food poisoning' refers to a sharp outbreak of illness, often affecting more than one individual, shortly after a meal. Non-bacterial causes include metallic poisoning (from utensils used for food storage or cooking) and certain fungi. Bacterial food poisoning is caused by those serotypes of *Salmonella* that are primarily parasites of animals (examples are *S. typhimurium, hadar, enteritidis* and *heidelberg*) and certain other organisms such as *Staphylococcus aureus* and *Clostridium welchii*. In the majority of cases the illness is unpleasant but brief. A permanent carrier state is rare.

Epidemiology

The causative organisms are widely distributed in the animal kingdom. Some tend to restrict themselves to geographical areas, although the prevalence of particular serotypes is constantly changing. *S. typhimurium* is the commonest cause of human salmonella infection in Europe and America.

Human infections are acquired mainly from cattle, pigs, poultry and eggs, although other sources have also been implicated, e.g. milk, shellfish and petfoods. Transmission is normally due to organisms surviving in undercooked meat, or by cooked meat becoming contaminated by infected meat or a human carrier. They need sufficient time at a suitable temperature to multiply. The organisms survive deep freezing.

In Britain, the incidence (judged by notification rates) has increased since

1972 as a result of a rise in salmonella food poisoning; this is believed to be because of the intensive rearing of poultry and an increase in poultry meat production. Outbreaks in hospitals, especially in children's wards, are common; infection spreads directly from child to child or by way of staff.

Prevention

Transmission of the organisms may follow a long and complicated path involving animal feedstuffs, the farm, market, abattoir, cold storage, shop and kitchen. Bacterial contamination may occur at any stage in this chain and preventive measures therefore need to be applied in a wide variety of settings. Improved animal husbandry to reduce the prevalence of infection in animals, hygienic production and distribution of food, and health education to achieve high standards of food preparation are all essential measures. Of particular importance is the need to destroy organisms by heat (after adequate thawing if the meat is frozen) and to protect cooked food from contamination.

BOVINE TUBERCULOSIS

The primary lesion in infection by *Mycobacterium bovis* is situated in the tonsil or Peyer's patches, with spread to the cervical or mesenteric lymph glands.

Epidemiology

The disease has been largely eradicated in Briatin but is still common in developing countries. It is transmitted by milk from infected cows.

Prevention

Control of the source of infection is by tuberculin testing of cattle and slaughter of infected animals. Transmission is prevented by pasteurization of milk; in Britain only 5% of milk is sold untreated.

BRUCELLOSIS

Brucellosis is an infection caused by organisms belonging to the genus *Brucella*. The name commemorates the work of David Bruce who in 1877 isolated the organism from four patients who had died in Malta of 'Mediterranean Fever'.

Epidemiology

It is primarily a disease of animals, especially of cattle (*Br. abortus* being most commonly involved), goats (always *Br. melitensis*), sheep (usually *Br.*

melitensis) and pigs (*Br. suis*). Man becomes infected in two ways: by drinking infected milk or its products and by contact with infected animals.

Br. melitensis is the cause of the disease in Malta and most of the Mediterranean countries. When cases of *Br. melitensis* infection occur in Britain, the organism has almost always been acquired abroad.

Brucellosis due to *Br. abortus* or *Br. suis* is largely an occupational disease affecting men, especially veterinary surgeons, dairy farmers and abattoir workers. Each time an infected cow calves, the attendant is sprayed with the organisms and infection takes place by way of the skin, mucous membranes and conjunctivae or by inhalation. The number of cases acquired in Britain has declined enormously as a result of compulsory eradication schemes for cattle and legislation under which untreated milk that is sold must be from brucella-accredited herds.

Prevention

Serological tests in cattle are reliable indicators of infection; in Britain infected animals are slaughtered. Calves are immunized but eradication measures are much more difficult to achieve with goats, sheep or pigs. The other important methods of prevention are pasteurization of milk (from cows and goats) and the wearing of protective clothing by veterinary surgeons and abattoir workers. The milk ring test is a sensitive indicator of brucellae in cows' milk.

HYDATID DISEASE

In man, hydatid disease is caused by infection with tapeworm larvae of the genus *Echinococcus*. There are two important species: *E. granulosus* and *E. multilocularis*. *Echinococcus* produces hydatid cysts, usually in the liver, but occasionally also in the lungs or other organs.

Epidemiology

Hydatid disease occurs worldwide. It is most common in those countries devoted to sheep-rearing. In Britain, the incidence is highest in the rural areas of Wales.

Dogs become infected by eating the viscera of sheep containing hydatid cysts. The worms develop in the dog's small intestine and its infected faeces contaminate grass and farmland. Man becomes infected by handling the dogs and by eating contaminated garden produce. Because of these occupational factors, most cases occur in men. Elsewhere in the world, other animals (wild dingos, wallabies, wolves, foxes, voles, etc.) act as hosts.

Prevention

Infected meat should be condemned, whether intended for human or animal consumption. Only cooked meat should be used for dog food. Farmers and shepherds should be informed about the dangers of too close an association with dogs. Dogs should be dewormed regularly. Good animal husbandry, with slaughter under controlled conditions in abattoirs, is important. Dead intermediate hosts should be incinerated or buried deeply.

ASCARIS (ROUNDWORM) AND TAENIA (TAPEWORM) INFECTIONS

Roundworm infection is caused by the nematode *Ascaris lumbricoides*. When the eggs are swallowed, larvae are liberated in the small intestine from whence they are carried to the lung through the bloodstream. From the lung they migrate via the trachea to the intestine where they develop into adult worms. Tapeworm infection is caused by the cestodes *Taenia saginata* and *Taenia solium*. When larvae are swallowed, the cysticercus is liberated in the small intestine where the adult develops. The larval stage of *T. solium* can live in human tissues, such as the brain or muscles.

Epidemiology

Roundworm infection occurs throughout the world but especially in tropical Africa and the Far East. The prevalence of infection is high in regions where defaecation occurs in the open, leading to contamination of soil and vegetables. Man becomes infected by swallowing the eggs in water or on contaminated vegetables.

Tapeworm infection is particularly common in tropical Africa and the Middle East. It is acquired by eating undercooked infected meat from the cow (*T. saginata*) or pig (*T. solium*).

Prevention

Since roundworm infection is soil transmitted, personal hygiene and sewage disposal are important. In endemic areas, human faeces should not be used as soil fertilizer (except after composting), and defaecation in the open should not be permitted.

Tapeworm infections can be prevented by cooking meat thoroughly so that any cysts are killed. Meat inspection and animal hygiene are important preventive measures.

4

Percutaneous infections and diseases transmitted by direct contact

Pathogenic organisms may enter the body through the skin as a result of *insect bites* (examples are filariasis, leishmaniasis, malaria, trypanosomiasis and yellow fever), *animal bites* (rabies), *abrasions* (anthrax, leptospirosis and typhus), *wounds* (surgical wound infection and tetanus), *penetration* (schistosomiasis) or *injection* (hepatitis B).

Organisms may also enter the body as a result of *direct contact*, e.g. facial herpes, sexually transmitted diseases (including the majority of acquired immune deficiency syndrome cases), scabies and trachoma. Several of the communicable diseases considered in earlier chapters can be spread by direct contact with a case or carrier; examples are influenza and glandular fever.

FILARIASIS

Filarial nematodes cause several diseases in man, including Bancroft's filariasis (due to *Wuchereria bancrofti*), Malayan filariasis (due to *W. malayi*) and onchocerciasis (due to *Onchocerea volvulus*).

Epidemiology

It is estimated that well in excess of 250 million people in the tropics are infected with filarial nematodes. The greatest number of cases of Bancroft's filariasis is in India but the disease is also found in many other Asian countries, in Africa and in Central and South America. The parasite affects whole communities and is characteristically found on the hot, humid coastal plains and in the insanitary slums of overpopulated cities. In chronic cases the most common complication is hydrocoele; elephantiasis is a less common complication.

In areas of high transmission nearly all the people may be infected. In the worst affected areas, the prevalence of blindness (due to microfilariae entering the eye) may be as high as 30%. This 'river blindness' can disrupt socioeconomic life, forcing people to move from their villages and set up elsewhere, often on less fertile land.

34

The microfilariae of Bancroft's or Malayan filariasis are spread by many species of mosquito. The main reservoir of infection is man. A high proportion of infections may be clinically silent but these cases are capable of spreading the disease. Onchocerciasis is transmitted by the bite of the female blackfly of the genus *Simulium* which breeds in the highly oxygenated water of hillside streams or in large rivers below cataracts.

Prevention

Control measures are directed against the parasite in man and against the vector insect. Treatment (for example with diethylcarbamazine) is usually effective in destroying most of the microfilariae, and mass campaigns have been successfully carried out in many countries. Vector control is by the use of insecticides and the elimination of breeding places. Visits to endemic areas should be avoided; if unavoidable, protective clothing should be worn.

LEISHMANIASIS

Protozoan parasites of the genus *Leishmania* cause a disease in man that ranges from self-healing cutaneous lesions to disseminated, often fatal, visceral infections.

Epidemiology

The parasites are widely distributed in Africa, Asia, Europe and Central and South America. Animal reservoirs of infection include rodents and other small mammals and the canine species; man may sometimes be the main reservoir. Transmission is by the bite of infected female sandflies. Skin tests show that in some areas over 90% of the population have been infected.

Visceral leishmaniasis occurs widely throughout the Old and New Worlds. The 'infantile' type occurs predominantly in children under the age of 5 years; dogs and other wild canine speices provide the reservoir. Kala-azar occurs in the north-eastern parts of the Indian subcontinent; widespread spraying programmes as part of the malaria control programmes in the 1950s led to the virtual disappearance of the disease in India, but the cessation of spraying in the mid-1970s was followed by a serious epidemic. It occurs mainly in young adult males. Man is the only known reservoir. In East Africa, leishmaniasis is a disease of arid, often sparsely populated, marginal lands. Substantial outbreaks have occurred, usually affecting children. Sporadic cases are usually in young adult males.

The characteristic lesion of cutaneous leishmaniasis is a chronic ulcerating lesion, the 'Oriental sore'. There is also a diffuse form of the disease which is commonly confused with leprosy; sometimes the disease invades the mucocutaneous regions.

Prevention

Vector control by insecticide spraying is the only method of prevention at present.

MALARIA

Malaria is an infection caused by parasites of the genus *Plasmodium*. The species infecting man are *P. vivax*, *P. falciparum*, *P. malariae* and *P. ovale*. *P. falciparum* causes a more serious illness ('malignant malaria') than the other varieties. The only certain proof of infection is the finding of malarial parasites in the blood. The disease has serious economic consequences in the areas involved.

Epidemiology

The global situation is depressing; around 12 million new cases are reported to the World Health Organization each year, half being in African countries south of the Sahara. Malaria kills around 1 million infants and children each year; there is also the growing problem of drug-resistant strains of *P. falciparum*. Following successful eradication measures in many countries, the disease has made a remarkable comeback, especially in Asia and some parts of Central and South America. In tropical Africa, the impact of control measures has been minimal partly because of the resistant nature of the vector.

When malaria occurs in Britain, it is in immigrants who have visited their relatives in the tropics or who are newly arrived, in businessmen or technologists working in malarious areas and in holidaymakers. The majority of imported cases are due to *P. vivax*.

The classic manner of contracting malaria is by the bite of the female anopheline mosquito. It can be acquired at relatively short stops on a journey, for example while refuelling an aeroplane.

Prevention

Antimalarial chemoprophylaxis will prevent infection in the majority of cases but it does not provide an absolute guarantee of protection. It must be taken when visiting any area where malaria might be acquired and continued for an absolute minimum of 4 weeks, and preferably 6 weeks, after leaving the endemic area. Children of all ages and pregnant women require antimalarial drugs but certain of them are contraindicated. The most important methods of vector control are house spraying to kill the adult mosquito and drainage of waters where the mosquito breeds. Repellant creams and mosquito nets also play some part in preventing infection.

Reasons for the failure of control programmes include the emergence of resistant strains, financial constraints, lack of government commitment, the rising cost of insecticides and transport, and population movements of nomads and workers.

TRYPANOSOMIASIS

There are two forms of trypanosomiasis: African trypanosomiasis ('sleeping sickness'), caused by *Trypanosoma gambiense* (in West and Central Africa) or *T. rhodesiense* (in East Africa); and American trypanosomiasis (Chagas' disease), caused by *T. cruzi*.

Epidemiology

African trypanosomiasis occurs in 100–200 distinct foci scattered over the tsetse belt of Africa. Man is the principal host but *T. rhodesiense* can also parasitize certain species of wild game. The disease is transmitted by the bite of *Glossina* (tsetse fly). The disease is confined to countries lying between latitude 10°N and 25°S, and an estimated 50 million people are at risk.

Chagas' diseases is transmitted by bloodsucking bugs which occur naturally in the area extending from 200 miles south of New York to Southern Argentina. In rural areas most houses have bug infestation and, when families move to towns in search of work, they often take bugs on their baggage and trypanosomiasis in their blood. WHO once estimated that 7 million people were infected but this is an underestimate today; in Brazil alone, 6 million people are infected.

Prevention

Because of the vastness of the area that belongs to the tsetse fly, the task of eradicating African trypanosomiasis is daunting. It involves insecticide spraying, game extermination, bush clearing and concentrating the people to such a density that their agricultural and other activities eradicate the tsetse fly's habitats. Reservoirs of infection are also reduced by surveying infected communities and treating all those found to be infected. Chemoprophylaxis has a role in the control of *T. gambiense* infections. The control of Chagas' disease relies on insecticide spraying and health education.

YELLOW FEVER

This is one of the arbovirus infections. Typical cases carry a very high fatality but serological surveys have shown that the disease may also exist in a mild or symptomless form.

Epidemiology

The disease is endemic in tropical Africa and in South and Central America. Although all ages are susceptible, infants under 6 months are rarely affected.

Yellow fever is a disease of monkeys, and it is transmitted by mosquitoes such as *Aedes aegypti*. A high average temperature is necessary for the viral stage in the mosquito.

Prevention

Immunization with a live attenuated virus protects for at least 10 years. An international certificate of vaccination against yellow fever becomes valid 10 days after vaccination and remains valid for 10 years. In cases of revaccination, the certificate becomes valid immediately. The other method of prevention is the eradication of mosquitoes.

RABIES

Rabies is due to a virus of the rhabdovirus group. Although the incubation period is usually 2–6 weeks, it may vary from 10 days to 2 years. Hydrophobia (the fear of drinking) is a well-known feature of the disease. Fatality is 100% unless early protection is given after exposure, but before symptoms develop.

Epidemiology

Except for a few countries, such as Britain and Scandinavia, rabies is widely prevalent among animals throughout the world. The disease is transmitted to man by the bite of an infected animal, particularly a dog, fox, wolf or bat. Three-quarters of cases are due to dog bites, and the animal usually dies within a few days. There is also a risk of infection from being scratched by a rabid animal.

Human rabies has not occurred in Britain for several decades, but the spread of the disease in many parts of Europe is a matter for concern. In Central Europe, where the fox is the main vector, failure of control has been due to inadequate measures to reduce the fox population.

Prevention

Freedom from rabies in Britain depends on the policy of 6 months' quarantine for all imported canine animals. Prophylactic immunization (with human diploid cell vaccine) is recommended for all persons exposed in the course of their work to special risks of contracting the disease.

When a person has been bitten by a suspected rabid animal, the wound should be cleaned and irrigated, antiserum administered (injecting some around the wound) and active immunization begun. Travellers should be educated to seek local medical help without delay if they are bitten, scratched or licked by animals.

The English Channel will prove an adequate barrier to the reintroduction of rabies provided the UK animal import and quarantine regulations are not broken.

ANTHRAX

Anthrax is a naturally occurring disease of sheep and cattle. Occasionally man acquires the infection through contact with animals or their products. The most common manifestation is a cutaneous necrotic lesion. The causative organism is an anaerobic spore-forming bacterium, *Bacillus anthracis*.

Epidemiology

Anthrax is no longer a serious health problem in developed countries but it remains fairly common among some cattle-rearing tribes in the tropics. Spores are formed when bacilli are shed from the saliva, faeces and urine of the dying animal host. They remain viable in soil for many years and will germinate when ingested by animals. Human infection may be acquired from the sick animal, from its contaminated environment (hay, straw, sacking) or from animal products (hides, bones). Crushed bones from India and Pakistan are a danger to workers manufacturing glue, gelatine, bone-meal and fertilizers. Contaminated hides present a hazard to dock and tannery workers. The organism enters the body through skin abrasions. A severe intestinal form of the disease may result from eating the meat of an infected animal. 'Wool sorter's disease', due to the inhalation of spore-laden dust, was at one time common in the woollen industry; it carried a high fatality.

Prevention

In Britain, anthrax is uncommon among animals; when it does occur the animal is killed and the carcass is disposed of by cremation or deep burial in lime, without necropsy. Animals in the herd are immunized and all animal movements are prohibited.

Workers at risk should be immunized against the disease and provided with protective clothing. Buildings where imported animal products are processed should be properly ventilated; extractor fans and ample washing facilities are obligatory.

LEPTOSPIROSIS

Leptospirosis is an acute infection caused by a genus of small spirochaetes known as *Leptospira*. Approximately 150 serotypes of pathogenic leptospiras are recognized but only two (*canicola* and *icterohaemorrhagiae*) cause disease in Britain.

Epidemiology

Leptospirosis has a worldwide distribution. It occurs wherever there is contact with infected wild and domestic animals or their excretions. It is most prevalent in the rice fields of Italy and Spain. The main animal reservoir for the *canicola* serogroup (causing canicola fever) is the dog; for the *icterohaemorrhagiae* serogroup (causing Weil's disease), rats, dogs and pigs.

Human infection results from direct contact with the urine or tissues of an infected animal or indirectly from contaminated water or soil. Infection commonly takes place by way of moist or abraded skin, mucous membranes and conjunctivae. Individuals at risk include sewer workers, abattoir workers, coalminers, farmers, fish workers and those employed on canals, docks and river drainage. Infection via the conjunctiva follows swimming or accidental immersion in contaminated waters. In the home, pet dogs can transfer the disease to children and adults through their infected urine. Laboratory workers are at risk from handling animals and from inoculation of infected materials.

Prevention

Sewermen, canal workers and abattoir workers should wear protective clothing and those individuals at risk who have cuts or abrasions should receive prophylactic penicillin. In hazardous occupations, immunization with local serogroups has proved of value. Rodents in warehouses, grain stores, sugar plantations and rice fields should be eradicated where possible, and it is essential that infected premises are disinfected with hypochlorite solution. Immunization of domestic animals is said to afford a high degree of protection against leptospirosis but it will not prevent the development of the carrier state when infection occurs. Intramuscular streptomycin is effective in the treatment of animal carriers.

THE TYPHUS FEVERS

The typhus fevers are caused by species of rickettsial organisms, for example *R. prowazeki* (causing epidemic typhus), *R. mooseri* (murine typhus) and *R. rickettsi* (Rocky Mountain spotted fever).

Epidemiology

These diseases are transmitted by arthropods — the louse, rat flea, tick and mite.

Louse-borne (epidemic) typhus infects only man. Endemic foci exist in Central and Eastern Africa and in South America. Human infection results from contamination of skin abrasions with louse faeces. It is endemic where man lives in overcrowded, unhygienic, lice infested conditions, and explosive epidemics occur.

Murine typhus is a rodent infection; it exists throughout the world and is conveyed to man by the faeces of infected rat fleas.

Tick-borne typhus is primarily a disease of animals, e.g. rodents in the case of Rocky Mountain spotted fever, but it may occur sporadically in man.

Scrub typhus is transmitted by the larvae of certain mites. It is a rural disease and is distributed in a triangular area bounded by Japan, West Pakistan and Australia. Scrub typhus was a serious problem to troops during World War II and the Vietnam War.

Prevention

Control of the vectors involves the use of insecticides to kill lice (on the skin and clothes), ticks (on dogs) and mites (on the skin and in the surface soil). Spotted fever and scrub typhus cannot be prevented by vector control since the widespread occurrence of the vectors would require treatment of enormous areas. Chemoprophylaxis protects against scrub typhus.

SURGICAL WOUND INFECTION

Joseph Lister believed that surgical wound sepsis was caused by air-borne organisms and introduced the use of carbolic acid dressings in an attempt to kill any bacteria that had already reached the wound. Later, his operations were carried out under a phenol spray in the hope of killing any bacteria yet to be introduced into the wound. Much of the Listerian technique gave way to the 'aseptic' school of surgery and it was realized that bacteria were transferred to other patients from septic wounds on the surgeon's hands or by his instruments. The measures introduced by Lister and his successors brought about a great reduction in postoperative wound sepsis but there remained a residue of hospital-acquired infection which, although mild by comparison with the terrible sepsis and gangrene of the pre-Lister era, were bad enough to be disturbing. With the introduction of antibiotics came the hope that bacterial infections might be completely controlled, but it was later realized that the incidence of some antibiotic-resistant infections had actually increased.

An investigation of over 3000 surgical operations in 21 different hospitals in the UK showed that 10% of the wounds were affected by some postoperative sepsis and yielded pathogenic bacteria on culture, but the sepsis rate varied widely in different hospitals. Some operations, such as colostomy and breast operations, were found to have much higher sepsis rates than others, e.g. orthopaedic. *Staphylococcus aureus* was the commonest pathogen but infections with coliform organisms were also common, particularly after operations in the abdominal cavity. The sepsis rates reported in that study probably underestimate the magnitude of the problem since certain operations (surgery of the lower urinary tract) were excluded.

While there is some evidence that wound sepsis (i.e. the presence of suppuration) arises from organisms acquired in the wards, there is much to support the view that often it is attributable to organisms introduced into the wound at the time of operation. This is certainly true of much sepsis due to Gram-negative organisms following the opening of the bowel or urinary tract. The failure of technique about which there is little dispute is poor haemostasis leading to haematoma. The site of the wound is also of importance, e.g. in surgery for varicose veins, wounds in the groin become infected more frequently than wounds in the leg made at the same operation. This may well relate to the bacterial population of the adjacent perineum. The use of drains to remove fluid from body cavities is also associated with a high incidence of sepsis in the wound.

Before positive pressure ventilation was provided in operating theatres, air was often being sucked into the operating theatre from the rest of the hospital, resulting in high bacterial air counts and consequent high wound sepsis rates. In addition to this evidence, there are many reports of sepsis attributable to operating theatre staff who were *Staphylococcus* carriers or who had septic lesions. Some people (patients and staff) disseminate large numbers of staphylococci into the air. Within a week of admission to hospital, 38% of patients carry hospital staphylococci in the nares and 7% develop wound infection of the same type.

Several factors have been found to be independently associated with an increased risk of postoperative sepsis, namely age over 60, male sex, long duration of operation, incision over 6 inches (150 cm) and insertion of a drain.

Prevention

A wide spectrum of measures is required to maintain a low level of postoperative infection. The number of organisms on the patient's skin can be greatly reduced by adequate preparation involving washing and the application of antiseptics. Pre- and postoperative patients with infections should be isolated and infected wounds should be covered to reduce the spread of the infecting bacteria. Indiscriminate use of antibiotics should be avoided in order to prevent the emergence of resistant strains in the hospital environment. Strict aseptic techniques must be established in the ward and operating theatre, and all personnel with established staphylococcal infections excluded from the surgical ward and operating theatre. The preparation of the hands of operating staff includes the use of anitbacterial agents such as chlorhexidine or hexachlorophene. Positive pressure ventilation in the theatre should ensure that it is like an oasis in the desert. No-one should enter the operating theatre without removing street clothing and donning an operating suit, mask and shoes. Traffic in the operating theatre should be minimized and purposeful.

TETANUS

'*Tetanos*' (Greek) means tension and the lay name 'lock jaw' describes one of its manifestations. The disease, caused by a powerful neurotoxin produced by *Clostridium tetani*, is characterized by muscular rigidity with superimposed spasms.

Epidemiology

Spores of *Cl. tetani* are present in the faeces of herbivorous animals, especially horses, and they are ubiquitous in dust and soil. Any damage to skin or mucous membranes may admit spores to the underlying tissues. They germinate only under strictly anaerobic conditions, and the wounds most likely to engender tetanus are those that are deep, contaminated with soil or a foreign body, complicated by vascular damage, or for which treatment is delayed more than about 6 hours. In tropical countries, neonatal tetanus is common because of the practice of covering the umbilical stump with mud or dung; it carries a very high fatality (80–90%).

Annual world mortality from tetanus may be as high as 2 million with an average case fatality of 50%. Most of these deaths are from neonatal tetanus. With the virtual disappearance of horses from our roads and the introduction of immunization, tetanus has become a rare disease in Britain. People under 50 and men who fought in the second World War are those most likely to have been immunized. Soldiers are particularly exposed to infection but in Britain most recent cases have been in agricultural workers, elderly gardeners and young sportsmen. In developing countries, the majority of cases are under 10 years of age.

Prevention

The aim should be to immunize the entire community with tetanus toxoid and to ensure a protective level of antibodies throughout life. The primary course is given in infancy, with booster doses at school entry and when an injury is sustained. Active immunization should also be given to high-risk groups such as military personnel, nurses and, in developing countries, women (to prevent puerperal and neonatal tetanus).

In the unimmunized person, no wound is too trivial to cause tetanus and active immunization should be started. It should also be started if the patient is not known to be immune, if treatment has been delayed or if the wound is septic or heavily contaminated. If the patient is known to be immune, the policy will depend on the nature of the injury. Normally, a toxoid booster is given, provided no dose has been given within the previous year; for many minor injuries a toxoid booster will not be given provided the patient has had a full primary course and the last booster is within 5 years. All wounds must be thoroughly cleaned, and foreign matter and necrotic tissue removed. Although *Cl. tetani* spores are not killed by antibiotics, penicillin or tetracycline are used to kill the vegetative forms of the organism.

The number of spores is reduced in operating theatres and central sterile supply departments by air filtration and the use of antiseptics on walls and floors. Spores are destroyed on surgical instruments and dressings by gamma-irradiation or autoclaving; heat-sensitive instruments are decontaminated by soaking in a mixture of methanol and sodium hypochlorite.

In tropical countries, health education about the proper care of the umbilical stump is essential if neonatal tetanus is to be prevented.

SCHISTOSOMIASIS (BILHARZIA)

Schistosomiasis is a group of diseases caused by trematodes of the genus *Schistosoma*. The three most common species to infect man are *S. haematobium*, *S. mansoni* and *S. japonicum*. *S. haematobium* commonly infects the vesical plexus of the bladder, and *S. mansoni* and *S. japonicum* the branches of the mesenteric veins.

Epidemiology

Probably around 200 million people are infected with schistosomiasis; the disease is common in Africa and the Middle East (*S. haematobium* and *S. mansoni*), Central and South America (*S. mansoni*) and the Far East (*S. japonicum*). It is predominantly an infection of agricultural and rural communities. Inadequate sewage disposal (leading to water pollution) and urination into water supplies are potent factors in its transmission. New irrigation schemes, such as in the Nile delta, and man-made lakes have led to increased spread in some areas. It is an occupational hazard for fishermen, peasant farmers and agricultural workers in developing countries.

The parasites develop in certain snails; man acquires the infection by close contact with water, i.e. wetting the skin or mucous membrane of the mouth with water containing infective larvae (cercariae) shed by the snail hosts. The cercariae penetrate the skin to enter a further development in the liver and portal venous system. The adult female lays eggs which are voided in the urine or faeces. Most infected individuals harbour few parasites but a small proportion are heavily infected and are responsible for excreting the bulk of the eggs; the heavy excretors are usually children.

Prevention

Control measures are directed towards (1) reducing the snail population by means of molluscicides and improved irrigation practices; and (2) reducing the egg output using schistosomacides. Many patients with low rates of egg excretion have severe lesions; it is therefore desirable to treat all infected individuals to achieve maximum disease control, but particularly important to ensure that heavy excretors are treated. Progress has been slow where schistomiasis control programmes have not been accorded appropriate priority in public health programmes. The provision of fresh water supplies for washing, drinking and toilet facilities will reduce the incidence of schistosomiasis.

HEPATITIS B (SERUM HEPATITIS)

This was formerly known as 'homologous serum jaundice'. It is caused by a small virus and has an incubation period of 40–160 days. Severity ranges from clinically inapparent cases to fulminating fatal cases. The virus is present in the blood during the incubation period and the acute phase of the disease, and also in 'silent' healthy carriers. Infection with the virus may progress to chronic liver disease and predisposes to the development of primary hepatocellular carcinoma.

Epidemiology

About 200 million people are thought to carry heptatitis B virus. The disease is transmitted by blood or blood products (or occasionally other body fluids such as saliva and semen), instruments contaminated with blood or, in drug addicts and during tattooing, by the repeated use of unsterilized needles. Outbreaks of serum hepatitis have occurred in some haemodialysis units among both patients and staff. A major reservoir of the disease exists in male homosexuals.

Carriers can be detected by the test for Australia antigen which is positive in about 0.1% of the population in north-west Europe and North America, but much more often (up to 5%) in tropical countries and as high as 15–30% in the Far East.

Prevention

The prevention of serum hepatitis depends primarily on the screening of blood donations and the identification of infected persons, including carriers, and their exclusion from the panel of blood donors. They should also be excluded from haemodialysis units and should instead be dialysed at home. Appropriate precautions (rubber gloves, disposable syringes) must be taken by staff working in dialysis units or caring for hepatitis B patients.

Safe transmission of all blood specimens to laboratories is important. If not disposable, every piece of apparatus that pierces the skin (needles, transfusion sets, lancets) should be sterilized by heat or ethylene oxide.

Passive immunization using hepatitis B immunoglobulin is indicated when blood or other material containing hepatitis B surface antigen is accidentally inoculated, ingested or splashed on the conjuctiva. The results of trials of active immunization using hepatitis B surface antigen are promising and the vaccine is available in limited quantities for use in selected groups such as drug addicts, male homosexuals and those in high-risk occupations. Attempts are in progress to reduce the incidence of neonatal infection by the use of immunoglobulin followed by active immunization.

Hepatitis B is a notifiable disease; this procedure initiates the investigation of links between cases, possible sources of infection and means of transmission.

NON-A/NON-B HEPATITIS

This illness is generally mild and often subclinical but it may be followed by prolonged viraemia and a persistent carrier state. Evidence points to the existence of at least two causative viruses.

Epidemiology

In some parts of the world, this is the most common form of hepatitis occurring after blood transfusion and the administration of certain plasma derivatives. It has also occurred in haemodialysis and renal transplantation units and among drug addicts.

Prevention

The measures are those described for hepatitis B.

SEXUALLY TRANSMITTED DISEASES

These diseases include syphilis (caused by *Treponema pallidum*), gonorrhoea (*Neisseria gonorrhoeae*), herpes genitalis and non-specific infections.

Epidemiology

It is estimated that about 200 million new cases of gonorrhoea and 40 million new cases of syphilis occur in the world each year — and these are probably underestimates. It is difficult to compare the incidence of sexually transmitted diseases between countries because of differences in recording systems, but there are indications that they are much more common in the USA than in Britain.

In the UK there is a voluntary system of notification by STD clinics. Statistical information derived from these clinics underestimate the true prevalence of sexually transmitted disease because some patients are treated by their general practitioners, treat themselves with antibiotics, or have mild symptoms and do not seek treatment. The total number of new cases seen each year is now over half a million, of which a quarter are non-specific urethritis (the cause of which is uncertain).

Following a post-war peak, the incidence of syphilis declined rapidly and this has been attributed to the discovery and widespread use of penicillin and other antibiotics. An alarming increase in gonorrhoea (*Fig. 4.1*) and non-specific urethritis (*Fig. 4.2*) occurred in Britain during the 1960s; in recent years there has been a marked increase in incidence in homosexual men. Syphilis also increased in the 1960s and 1970s (*Fig. 4.3*). The old classical venereal diseases — syphilis, gonorrhoea and chancroid — now constitute

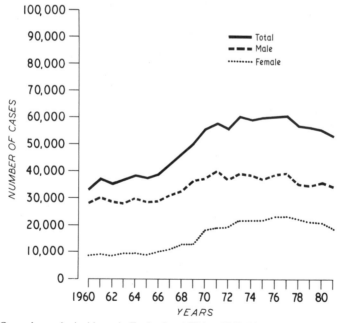

Fig. 4.1 Gonorrhoea: the incidence in England and Wales, 1960–81.

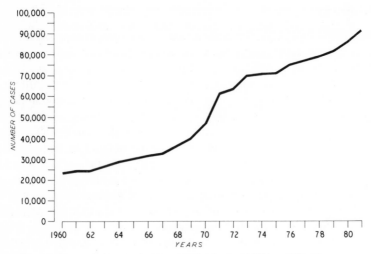

Fig. 4.2 Non-specific urethritis: the incidence in England and Wales, 1960–81.

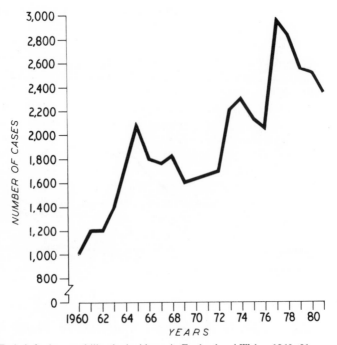

Fig. 4.3 Early infectious syphilis: the incidence in England and Wales, 1960–81.

only 16% of the workload of STD clinics and the increase in patients is the result of the newly recognized diseases including genital herpes and non-specific genital infections. The main reasons for these trends are: increasing promiscuity, male homosexuality, more population movement, failure to warn young people of the real danger, the use of oral contraceptives instead of barrier methods, the absence of symptoms in some 50% of cases of gonorrhoea in women, the short incubation period in gonorrhoea (3–5 days) and the emergence of penicillin-resistant strains of *N. gonorrhoeae*.

These infections cross all social barriers. High-risk groups include prostitutes, practising homosexuals, promiscuous young people, members of the armed forces and merchant seamen. The peak incidence is between 20 and 24 years, and in recent years there has been a marked increase in Britain in the number of infected girls aged 16 and 17.

Syphilis is almost always transmitted by sexual contact, whether normal, ano-genital or oral. Non-venereal transmission is unusual as the organism dies rapidly outside the body. The fetus may become infected *via* the maternal blood supply. Gonorrhoea is a highly infectious disease which, like syphilis, is almost always transmitted by sexual contact. It is believed that 10–20% of women develop salpingitis after a gonococcal infection but in some developing countries the prevalence of pelvic inflammatory disease is very high. Ophthalmia neonatorum results from infection of the infant during its passage down the birth canal. Within marriage, non-specific infections are more common than gonorrhoea.

Caused by herpes simplex virus (types 1 and 2), genital herpes is the fastest growing sexually transmitted disease in the UK. Current estimates put the number of people in the UK with genital herpes at about 200 000 with the number of new cases reported growing annually by more than 10%. In Britain, the incidence of genital herpes is now almost three times that of syphilis. The commonest mode of spread is by direct contact with infected secretions and it is likely that some cases of genital herpes are the result of oro-genital sexual practices. After the primary attack of genital herpes, the virus may assume an inactive state in the dorsal ganglia. Later it may reactivate and travel distally within the peripheral nerves to cause asymptomatic viral shedding or a clinical recurrence. The infection rate of neonates born to mothers excreting herpes virus late in pregnancy is around 50% but most escape significant disease. A link has been suggested between herpes simplex infection and carcinoma of the cervix but this is probably a non-specific indicator of sexual activity.

Prevention

The control of sexually transmitted disease depends on accurate diagnosis, effective treatment, careful follow-up, tracing of potentially infected contacts (those who are sources of infection and those who are secondarily infected) and health education directed at changing attitudes and behaviour. People who have symptoms need to come earlier for treatment and health education must emphasize the effectiveness of treatment. Congenital syphilis would be completely eliminated if antenatal tests for syphilis were always performed and the mother given appropriate treatment.

ACQUIRED IMMUNE DEFICIENCY SYNDROME

The widely accepted definition of this condition is as follows: A reliably diagnosed disease that is at least moderately indicative of underlying cellular deficiency (Kaposi's sarcoma in a patient aged less than 60 years or opportunistic infection) and where there is no known underlying cause of the cellular immune deficiency nor any other cause of reduced resistance reported to be associated with the disease. It is now well established that a retrovirus initially known as Lymphadenopathy Associated Virus (LAV) or Human T-cell Lymphotropic Virus type III (HTLV III) is the primary aetiological agent of AIDS. The generic Human Immunodeficiency Virus (HIV) is now used.

Other retroviruses in the group are known to cause leukaemia in animals and a human leukaemia case has recently been described, caused by HTLV IV.

Epidemiology

The first case of AIDS in the UK was reported in 1981 and serological studies as well as the epidemiology of AIDS indicate that HIV is probably a new infection in the Western World. There has been much speculation on its origin and the first cases retrospectively recognized as AIDS appeared in sub-Saharan Africa, especially Zaire. It has been suggested that the human infection was first derived by zoonosis from a closely related virus recently discovered in African green monkeys in which the virus appears to be non-pathogenic. In parts of Africa the disease has already reached epidemic proportions and is now doing so in the USA and Europe. Cases have been reported from almost 100 countries.

As in many virus diseases, infection with HIV has a wide spectrum of clinical expressions, from those individuals who are asymptomatic to the minority of people who are severely affected and develop AIDS. In a few patients a self-limiting glandular-fever-like illness — characterized by fever, macular rash and lymphadenopathy within a few days of infection — has been reported but in the majority of cases infection is probably unaccompanied by symptoms or signs. The incubation period between infection and development of AIDS is prolonged and has been found to vary between 15 months and 5 or more years. The signs of AIDS include insidious weight loss, malaise, fever and lymphadenopathy with the development of tumours (particularly Kaposi's sarcoma) and multiple opportunistic infections including *Pneumocystis carinii* pneumonia.

A number of syndromes such as Persistent Generalized Lymphadenopathy (PGL) and the AIDS-Related Complex (ARC) are features of HIV infection but falling short of the definition of AIDS. They are regarded as precursors to AIDS. Herpes zoster in an infected person is also a poor prognostic sign. To date, the cumulative fatality of AIDS is 100%.

The probability of persons infected with HIV developing AIDS is unknown. Current experience suggests that between 10% and 50% of cases progress to AIDS but, over 20 years or more, 100% progression is possible.

The epidemiological pattern of infection with HIV is similar to hepatitis B, being largely related to parenteral exposure to blood and blood products and to intimate (particulary sexual) contact. Groups at high risk for this infection currently include promiscuous homosexuals and bisexuals, intravenous drug abusers, patients with haemophilia (because of their treatment with Factor VIII) and sexual consorts of patients in these groups. By far the largest proportion has occurred in homosexual or bisexual men; the passive partners of anal intercourse are especially at risk. In Africa, and more recently in other countries, heterosexual intercourse is recognized as a principal vehicle of spread through the population.

Prevention

There are five prinicpal means of prevention:

1. *Surveillance* — National surveillance of AIDS in the UK is mainly dependent on confidential reporting of cases by clinicians to the Communicable Disease Surveillance Centre (and the equivalent Unit in Scotland). There is also a national collection of data on HIV infections.
2. *Counselling* — All individuals who are found to have positive antibody tests should receive counselling so that they understand the meaning of the results. Persons infected with HIV must not donate blood, body organs, other tissue or sperm. Because of the risk of infecting others by sexual intercourse, infected persons should be advised against multiple sexual partners and anal intercourse. Condoms may limit transmission of infection even in homosexuals. Although spread by saliva is unlikely, oral–genital contact should be avoided. Toothbrushes, razors and any other articles which could become contaminated with blood should not be shared. Skin piercing instruments, such as hypodermic needles, ear piercing equipment, tattoo and acupuncture needles, should be disposed of or autoclaved after use. In the event of an accident causing bleeding, the contaminated surfaces should be cleaned with household bleach freshly diluted 1 : 10 with water.

3. *Blood and blood products* — Persons with AIDS, groups at high risk of AIDS and their sexual contacts must not donate blood. Pooled factor VIII and Factor IX may transmit HIV but this risk is eliminated by heat treatment. In the UK all blood donations are now screened at Regional Blood Transfusion Centres for HIV antibody. People who believe themselves to be at risk of infection must not donate blood; this is crucial because even a reliable test cannot detect very early infections to which antibody response has not yet been generated. This 'window' lasts for an average of 3 months. In the UK, about one in a million units is infected. An antigen test is required to abolish the risk of transmission. In countries where screening of blood donors is not universal, tranfusion should be avoided if at all possible.
4. *Protection of health care staff* — The methods for protecting staff possibly exposed to infection from HIV are similar to the methods practised in the prevention of hepatitis B infection. This has included isolation nursing of patients with AIDS or symptomatic HIV infection (although the need for this is in doubt) and care with blood, needles, stool, urine and saliva. Pathology specimens should be kept to a reasonable minimum, collected with care and labelled 'high risk'. Postmortem examinations are in general not done on these patients and protective clothing is used when preparing infected dead bodies for disposal.

   Needlestick injuries carry a surprisingly low risk of infection.
5. *Education* — The public is being informed about the methods of spread of the disease and that the most effective control measure is the avoidance of promiscuous sexual behaviour, especially anal and unprotected intercourse. The dangers of sharing syringes and needles by drug abusers is also being emphasized and needle exchange schemes are being introduced to discourage shared use of 'equipment'.

The future

It has been estimated that up to one hundred thousand people may be infected with HIV in the UK in 1987 and one hundred million in the world. Using current prevalence, up to 10 000 cases of AIDS can be anticipated in the UK within five years. Although the measures now introduced will help limit the spread of HIV infection, they will not eradicate it and there is an urgent need for research into preventive and curative measures although the natural lability of HIV makes vaccine development difficult.

SCABIES

This is a condition, characterized by itching and a rash, due to burrowing into the skin by the mite *Sarcoptes scabiei.*

Epidemiology

It occurs worldwide and in recent years there has been a rapid rise in incidence in Britain. Transmission is by direct skin-to-skin contact. While burrowing, the female mite layes her eggs. Hatching occurs in 4 or 5 days and the larvae escape on the skin, some to be transferred to new hosts, some to perish and others to burrow and grow into adult mites.

Scabies is often introduced into households by schoolchildren, the commonest sources being friends and relatives outside the home.

Prevention

Control of the infestation depends on adequate treatment of cases with benzyl benzoate or other scabicide, contact tracing and in some circumstances mass inspection of, for example, soldiers and schoolchildren.

TRACHOMA

Trachoma is a granulomatous conjunctivitis of viral origin which causes severe scarring of the cornea and eyelids, often causing blindness.

Epidemiology

It has been estimated that 500 million people, or one-sixth of the world's population, are affected. The disease flourishes in countries where living standards and personal hygiene are poor. Flies are often responsible for transmitting the disease; eye-to-eye spread is by infected fingers or towels.

Prevention

Improvement of living standards, elimination of flies and health education to encourage personal hygiene (including daily washing of the eyes) will help to reduce the incidence of trachoma. Early treatment using topical antibiotics helps to reduce secondary infection and preserve sight. An effective vaccine is not yet available.

5

Diseases of the cardiovascular system

In developed countries, heart attacks and strokes kill as many people as all other causes of death combined (*Table 5.1*). But the work that arterial diseases creates for general practitioners is relatively small; for example only 10% of all consultations in the age group 45–54 years are due to this cause. This is because many of the victims die quickly or the treatment given is mainly in hospital.

RAISED ARTERIAL BLOOD PRESSURE

There is no dividing line in the frequency distribution curve of arterial pressure so that there is no clear demarcation of hypertensives from normotensives. In order to compare the prevalence in different populations it is useful to adopt criteria such as those suggested by the World Health Organization: hypertension is systolic 160+ mm Hg, diastolic 95+; borderline hypertension is systolic 140–149, diastolic 90–94. These criteria are not synonymous with the need for treatment. In patients with raised arterial blood pressure, both systolic and diastolic pressures are usually elevated. While a minority of cases are due to recognizable causes such as renal or endocrine disease, coarctation of the aorta or toxaemia of pregnancy, for the great majority (95%) no cause can be found and these cases are referred to as 'essential hypertension'.

Table 5.1 Causes of death in Britain

	Percentage	
Circulatory diseases	49.8	Ischaemic heart disease 26.9%
		Cerebrovascular disease 12.4%
Neoplasms	22.7	Trachea, bronchus, lung 6.1%
Respiratory diseases	14.0	
Injuries, poisonings	3.6	
Others	9.9	

Epidemiology

Life insurance statistics show that mortality rises steadily and markedly with increasing elevation of both systolic and diastolic pressures. The excess mortality in individuals with hypertension is primarily due to cardiovascular and renal diseases. The importance of high blood pressure is that it is a major factor associated with atherosclerosis and its complications, mainly coronary and cerebrovascular disease. The absolute risk of raised blood pressure is greater in men than in women, since men are more liable to develop coronary artery disease.

Mean arterial pressure rises with age. Before the age of 50, mean blood pressures vary little between the sexes; thereafter pressures are substantially higher in women than in men. About 5% of middle-aged adults have diastolic pressures of 110 mm Hg or more and a further 15% in the range 100–109 mm Hg. The prevalence of hypertension is highest in the poorer socioeconomic groups. A number of studies support the view that obesity plays a significant part in influencing the blood pressure level, but it probably accounts for only about 10% of the variance in blood pressure of the population. Fat young men are more likely than thin young men to become hypertensive as they grow older. Population studies have shown a positive correlation between salt intake and blood pressure.

Essential hypertension runs in families but this may be due to environmental factors. In multiracial communities, it is more common in black people than in whites and this is probably due to an increased genetic susceptibility. Black people also have higher death rates from hypertension-related conditions such as stroke and heart failure.

Prevention

Stroke, left ventricular failure, ruptured aorta, and renal and retinal damage can be almost eliminated by bringing diastolic pressures to about 80 mm Hg. There is also mounting evidence that mortality from coronary heart disease may be reduced by the control of high arterial pressure.

The effect of high systolic or diastolic pressure on mortality disappears over the age of 70 and there is little evidence either for or against intervention in elderly hypertensives in the absence of organ damage.

Under the age of 60, prophylactic blood pressure reduction is of proven benefit in both men and women with uncomplicated essential hypertension having a diastolic pressure consistently at 110 mm Hg or higher. Some would say that this level should be lower since a study of the treatment of hypertension in the diastolic range 90–104 mm Hg has shown, after 5 years of treatment, a fall of 20% in mortality from all causes, of 47% in mortality from myocardial infarction, and of 46% in mortality from stroke. Long-term treatment with antihypertensive drugs should be considered only when other measures have proved inadequate.

Studies have shown that only about half of all hypertensives have been diagnosed; of these only about half receive antihypertensive treatment, and of these only about half have adequate reduction of blood pressure. This is referred to as 'the rule of halves'. In Western countries about 85% of the population see a doctor at least once in 3 years. Most cases of hypertension would therefore be identified if all general practitioners used their normal consultations for case-finding ('opportunistic screening'). Doctors in other branches of medicine have the same responsibility and should inform the general practitioner of any abnormalities.

About 10–15% of the adult population have levels of blood pressure which are believed to justify treatment (diastolic 10 mm Hg and above) and a further 20% will need systematic follow-up for pressures in the 90–99 mm Hg range. The detection and treatment of obesity, and reduction in the population's salt intake, are further important preventive measures.

ISCHAEMIC HEART DISEASE

The World Health Organization has defined this as: 'The cardiac disability, acute or chronic, arising from reduction or arrest of the blood supply to the myocardium in association with disease processes in the coronary arteries.' Ischaemic heart disease may present in a symptomatic form (myocardial infarction, angina pectoris, cardiac arrhythmia) or it may be symptomless (an electrocardiographic diagnosis or sudden death).

Epidemiology

Ischaemic heart disease is the single largest cause of death in the UK, being responsible for a quarter of all deaths (*Table 5.1*). It is especially prevalent as a cause of death in middle-aged men, accounting in the age group 45–64 for 40% of deaths in men and 10% of deaths in women.

Coronary artery disease is not a new condition, but as a registered cause of death it has increased dramatically in both sexes throughout the present century. Rates in both males and females have remained fairly constant in Britain since 1979, but in the USA and Australia mortality rates have fallen in recent decades because, it is thought, of a fall in cigarette consumption, increased control of hypertension and changes in the composition of dietary fat.

Ischaemic heart disease mortality is higher in Britain than in most other countries of the world (*Fig. 5.1*). Japan and France have particularly low rates whereas Finland (especially North Karelia) has the highest. A World Health Organization study of 12 European cities showed that national differences in the frequency of attacks of coronary heart disease correspond closely

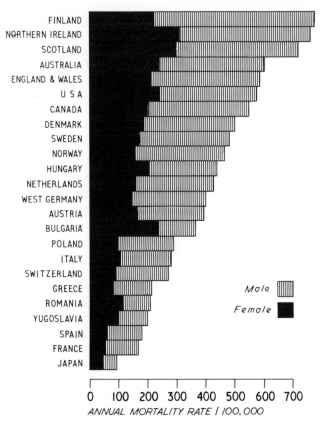

Fig. 5.1 Ischaemic heart disease mortality at ages 35–74 years in 1977 (standardized to the population of England and Wales).

with differences in the frequency of deaths from the disease. Within the UK, regional variations exist, with west central Scotland having a mortality rate which is almost double that in East Anglia. These differences persist after allowing for differences in the social class distribution. Differences in water hardness have been postulated as a cause for regional variations, since mortality tends to be highest in soft-water areas. Coronary heart disease is an uncommon condition in the less developed countries of the world and, where people have not come into close contact with 'civilization', it is virtually unknown.

Over the past three decades, the increase in ischaemic heart disease in males has been much greater than in females. This increase in males has been most marked in the age groups 35–44 years. There is a suggestion that the prevalence in this group has now begun to fall.

Death rates for coronary heart disease increase logarithmically with age

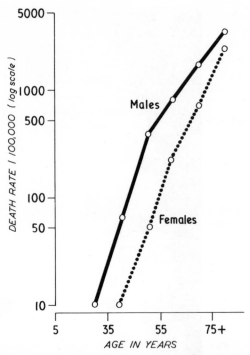

Fig. 5.2 Age-specific death rates in 1977 for ischaemic heart disease in England and Wales.

in both sexes (*Fig. 5.2*). At all ages they are higher for men than for women, e.g. a ratio of 3.5:1 at 55–64 years and 2.4:1 at 65–74 years.

Mortality is higher in social classes IV and V than in classes I and II; the gap between the classes is greatest for women and since 1951 it has been widening in both sexes.

Ischaemic heart disease is an important cause of morbidity as well as of mortality. In England and Wales it accounts for 8% of all working days lost because of ill health; 3–4% of men aged 45–64 years see their general practitioners each year on account of coronary heart disease.

Several risk factors have been identified; these are hypertension, raised serum total cholesterol and cigarette smoking. Many epidemiological studies have demonstrated the association between these factors and coronary heart disease, one of the best known and most expensive studies being that conducted in Framingham, a town near Boston in the USA. Five thousand adults aged 30–59 who were free of ischaemic heart disease were recruited in 1949 and studied at 2-yearly intervals. This and other studies have shown that, even allowing for the increase in blood pressure with age, the incidence of ischaemic heart disease rises steadily with increase in blood pressure (*Fig. 5.3*). Studies indicate that raised blood pressure is a risk factor independent

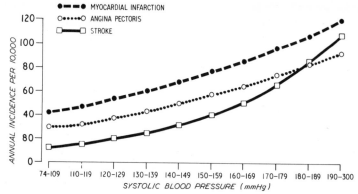

Fig. 5.3 Age-standardized incidence rate for myocardial infarction, angina pectoris and stroke at different levels of systolic blood pressure in men.

of the other factors such as smoking and blood cholesterol level. They also show a cumulative effect when more than one factor is present.

Cigarette smoking is a powerful and independent risk factor, particularly at younger ages. Pipe smokers are at slightly higher risk than non-smokers. There is evidence that it is the amount of smoke inhaled that is important rather than the form in which the tobacco is used. It promotes atheromatous and thrombotic changes in arteries and probably facilitates arrhythmias.

The pooled results of five American studies on men all initially free of signs of heart disease show that, of every three men who at the age of 40 were heavy smokers, one will have a major heart attack (probably fatal) before he reaches 65, compared with one out of seven non-smokers. The risk of coronary heart disease for smokers increases with the amount smoked, is detectable even among those smoking on average as few as 5–10 cigarettes a day and is four times as great (compared with non-smokers) for heavy smokers (40 cigarettes a day). It is reduced to not much more than the risk for lifelong non-smokers within a few years of giving up smoking. Autopsy studies have established that the amount and extent of coronary atheroma of people killed in accidents or dying from causes unrelated to smoking is directly proportional to how long and how much the deceased person had smoked. Smoking appears to have an important synergistic effect with the oral contraceptive pill, increasing the risk of coronary disease and subarachnoid haemorrhage.

The widening social class gap in mortality may be due to changes in smoking habits; the consumption in classes I and II has fallen relative to classes IV and V.

Countries which have a diet rich in fat are also those in which the death rate for coronary heart disease is high. International studies have shown that populations with high levels of serum cholesterol are those in which coronary death rates are high. Most of the cholesterol in the blood is manufactured by the body itself and is not derived from the diet. Prospective studies in developed countries have failed to show any association between individual fat intake and individual cholesterol levels. However, experiments have shown that raised blood cholesterol can be reduced by a reduction of total dietary fat, especially of saturated fatty acids. High density lipoprotein (HDL) has been thought to be related to atheroma and to coronary risk. However, recent research provides no evidence of it as an important risk factor. Less than 1% of hypercholesterolaemias are genetically determined. Homozygosity carries about 100% mortality by 60 years of age, mostly under the age of 30.

A study of London busmen showed a higher incidence of coronary heart disease among bus drivers than bus conductors; the heart disease also appeared earlier in the drivers and immediate mortality following a heart attack was higher. In a study of some 17 000 civil servants of all grades, it was found that there were fewer heart attacks among men who said they habitually engaged in vigorous exercise than in others. It is from such studies that the hypothesis has been derived that physical activity protects against ischaemic heart disease but we have to beware of the problems of self-selection in employment, i.e. that some of the people in light jobs may have taken those jobs because they are less physically fit or different in other ways. Confirmation of this was provided by the bus workers' study in which it was found that, even at the time of recruitment, drivers were taller, heavier and had a greater waist circumference and skinfold thickness than conductors and they also had higher mean blood pressure levels and higher serum cholesterol levels. However, their diets were very similar.

Before the menopause, the ratio of male to female death rates from ischaemic heart disease is about 6:1. Thereafter, it shows an abrupt decline which would be consistent with the sharp increase in risk affecting post-menopausal women. This relative immunity of women wears off whether the menopause occurs naturally or is artificially induced. Mean blood cholesterol is higher among women once they have passed the menopause.

Surveys from several parts of the world have shown that the incidence of heart attacks, as well as the death rate, has been increasing in recent years for women aged 35 and over. The first and by far the most important reason is cigarette smoking and the second, playing a minor role, is the increasing use of oral contraception. Over the age of 35, women on the pill have a slightly increased risk of coronary heart disease.

When all other risk factors are fully taken into account, obesity has little independent effect of the risk of arterial disease. Obesity expresses its effects through hyperlipidaemia, hypertension, the risks of diabetes, and perhaps reduced exercise.

The role of genetic factors in ischaemic heart disease is shown by twin studies and by the possible association with blood group O and the so-called

'Type A personality' (the ambitious, impatient and competitive members of society). Concordance rates of 26% have been reported in monozygotic twins and 14% in dizygotic twins; the difference is significant at the 5% level.

The fatality rate associated with heart attack is approximately 50%, with perhaps 60% of these deaths occurring within an hour, mainly outside the hospital and remote from resuscitation. Thus the opportunity for interference after an attack has begun is limited. Death has occurred in a third of attacks before a doctor can attend the patient and the use of a mobile team or training ambulance drivers has brought only marginal benefits.

Of all the risk factors discussed above, only smoking is a predictor of re-infarction.

Prevention

Probably about a half of all coronary deaths are preventable in our present state of knowledge. The most important known preventive measure is undoubtedly the control of smoking. Doll and Peto have shown that male doctors who stopped smoking between the ages of 34 and 55 reduced their mortality from coronary disease by half within 5 years, compared with doctors who continued to smoke. Over 55, the effect was much smaller. About half the eventual benefit on coronary mortality is reached 1 year after stopping.

Abnormalities of lipid metabolism are associated with an increased risk of arterial disease, and recent evidence suggests that changes in diet (reducing the amount of fat, especially fats rich in saturated fatty acids) can alter these risks. In particular, if all first-degree relatives (including children) of those developing coronary disease under the age of 50 were screened for blood fats, homozygosity might be identified and treated by arduous drug therapy and dietary control.

Physical activity is likely to be protective but the exercise needs to be taken regularly and often and to be strenuous enough to cause breathlessness and sweating. Heavy work for at least 30 minutes a day has been shown to improve the distribution of cholesterol fractions, to reduce the number of electrocardiographic abnormalities, systolic blood pressure and percentage body fat, and to improve glucose tolerance.

There is some evidence that the control of high blood pressure can be an important part of coronary disease prevention; the measures include weight reduction and lowering the salt intake, as well as the use of hypotensive drugs.

About two-thirds of any general practice population see their GP at least once a year and at least 90% consult in 5 years. A virtually complete ascertainment of major risk factors could be attained if consultations were designed to obtain this information and to record it in such a way that it could easily be acted upon, recalled, and not wastefully repeated.

The size of the water effect on mortality appears to be small compared with the effect of other risk factors; heavy smoking doubles the risk of a cardiovascular event, whereas soft water increases the risk by about 10%. There does not appear to be any justification for recommending water hardening.

The multifactorial nature of ischaemic heart disease has resulted in a move away from unifactorial intervention such as dietary change or smoking reduction. Community based projects — e.g. in North Karelia, Finland and in a WHO European collaborative trial — have demonstrated an important impact on lifestyles and shown that they might contribute to reduced rates of cardiovascular disease. However, it has not been easy to demonstrate clearly the effects of reducing risk factors in patients with moderate risk factor levels. A 'high-risk' strategy was initiated in the belief that those individuals with the highest levels of one or more risk factors were likely to show the greatest response to intervention. Most cases of ischaemic heart disease do not occur in the small number with high cholesterol levels; likewise it is those with only moderately raised levels of blood pressure who contribute most cases of ischaemic heart disease. It seems likely that the only approach that will be effective on a national basis is the population approach — health education and case-finding of those especially at risk.

Epidemiological studies are providing evidence that the place of treatment (whether at home, in an ordinary ward or in a coronary care unit) makes little difference to case fatality rates. For survivors, the risk of re-infarction is reduced if the patient gives up smoking.

RHEUMATIC HEART DISEASE

Rheumatic fever is a systemic febrile illness following a Group A beta-haemolytic streptococcal infection of the nasopharynx in a susceptible host. Rheumatic heart disease is the only significant complication of rheumatic fever.

Epidemiology

Normally, rheumatic fever follows only 0.3% of streptococcal infections, but during epidemics the rate increases ten-fold. The true incidence of rheumatic fever is unknown because attacks are often mild or subclinical. The prevalence in developed countries is 0.5 to 1 per thousand; in developing countries, rates ranging from 7 to 33 per thousand have been reported. Rheumatic carditis remains the most common cause of heart disease in developing countries but, in developed countries, the morbidity and mortality of rheumatic fever have been falling since the early part of the twentieth century due to an improvement in the standard of living and to a change in the prevalence and virulence of the organism. The apparent increase in the incidence of rheumatic fever in developing countries is ascribed to urbanization and the rapid increase in schooling, and also to an increased awareness of the disease, both by the patient and by the doctor.

Initial attacks seldom occur outside the 6–15 years age range; there is a peak in the incidence at 8 years. Susceptibility to recurrence continues to be relatively high until the third decade. There are no sex or racial differences in susceptibility. Evidence for a genetic susceptibility is provided by twin studies and by the higher incidence in the children of parents with rheumatic heart disease. Poor nutrition *per se* does not result in higher susceptibility; however, recent work suggests that inadequate nutrition in the first year of life may be significant. Poverty and overcrowding are important determinants of the disease, overcrowding probably being the more important. Epidemics are particularly likely to occur in institutions such as boarding schools and army camps.

Carditis occurs in about half the cases of rheumatic fever and 60% of these develop rheumatic heart disease. This figure is higher in developing countries. The average duration of the untreated attack is 3 months but, if severe carditis is present, the duration is often longer. Prior to the advent of antibiotics, about 70% of patients had one or more recurrences. Recurrence rates are highest in the first 3 years following the primary attack and significantly increase the morbidity and mortality from rheumatic heart disease. In untreated patients there is a mortality of 20% within 10 years.

Prevention

As it is impossible to make an accurate diagnosis of streptococcal pharyngitis clinically, a throat swab should be taken on presentation. Prompt treatment with penicillin (or erythromycin in penicillin-sensitive patients) prevents the development of rheumatic fever. Primary prevention is difficult in developing countries because patients with pharyngitis may not present for treatment, or facilities for culturing throat swabs may not be available.

Prevention of recurrent attacks is essential in all cases of rheumatic fever. Prophylaxis is by means of penicillin or sulphadiazine. The necessary duration is controversial, varying from 5 years after the last attack to continued prophylaxis for life.

STROKE (CEREBROVASCULAR ACCIDENT)

'Stroke' is defined as 'an episode of focal neurological dysfunction, with symptoms lasting more than 24 hours, due to a disturbance in the vascular supply to the brain'. It includes several clinical entities: cerebral haemorrhage, cerebral thrombosis, cerebral embolism and subarachnoid haemorrhage. The arbitrary limit of 24 hours is less important than the concept that transient ischaemic attacks are followed by full recovery of function.

Epidemiology

Atheroembolic brain infarction accounts for approximately 80% of all strokes, the remainder being due to haemorrhage. Clinically, it is difficult to distinguish infarction from haemorrhage, and death certification is notoriously inaccurate. Up to the age of 30 years, subarachnoid haemorrhage causes nearly half of all strokes; but after 30, other causes of stroke become progressively more common.

Fatality from stroke is about 60% by the end of the first month; in Britain cerebrovascular disease is only exceeded by cardiac disease and cancer as a cause of death. Each year, about 80 000 people in England and Wales die as a consequence of stroke. Local studies in England have shown that the incidence of stroke varies from 1.4 per thousand population in the south to 2.5 per thousand in the north where the prevalence is four times as great. Standardized mortality ratio for all forms of stroke is higher in the north and west of Britain than the south-east; it is highest in Scotland.

The incidence of stroke (apart from subarachnoid haemorrhage) rises steeply with age and is higher for males than for females. Stroke mortality in the USA and in the UK has shown a decline in all age groups between 35 and 74 years, particularly in women; the greatest decline has been in deaths from cerebral haemorrhage. Possible reasons for this include: change in death certification habits, lowered case fatality and improved treatment of hypertension. The incidence of first strokes has probably remained constant.

Stroke mortality for each pathological type is higher in social class V than in class I. Social class differences in mortality have widened rapidly since 1950, perhaps reflecting failure to deliver preventive care to poorer communities.

Epidemiological studies of the aetiology of stroke pose a number of difficulties. Case–control studies are often restricted to studying survivors (survival may itself be a function of certain risk factors); the level of a certain risk may change following a stroke (blood pressure is elevated for the first few days after a stroke); and prospective studies involve a long period of follow-up. The currently recognized risk factors (this does not necessarily imply a causal relationship) are: hypertension, diabetes mellitus, heart disease, transient ischaemic attacks and exogenous oestrogens.

Hypertension is the most important risk factor in cerebral infarction, cerebral haemorrhage and subarachnoid haemorrhage. There are several reports of a linear relationship between systolic and diastolic pressure and the risk of stroke in both sexes and at all ages. There is no critical level above which this operates, and it continues to operate after the first stroke. The higher levels of blood pressure among US black populations and their high risk of stroke are consistent with this relationship. There is considerable evidence to implicate salt consumption in the pathogenesis of hypertension and thereby of cerebrovascular disease. In Japan, where salt consumption is high, area mortality rates are closely related to the consumption of salt and of salty foods. Cerebral haemorrhage probably occurs more often in Japan than elsewhere. In England and Wales, where salt consumption is much lower, there is no such correlation.

When corrected for other major risk factors, the relative risk in diabetes is approximately two. An increased risk has also been shown to be associated with a variety of types of heart disease — left ventricular hypertrophy, ST abnormality, heart block, coronary artery disease, atrial fibrillation and congestive cardiac failure.

A previous history of stroke or transient ischaemic attack (TIA) makes the probability of a subsequent stroke high. In one cohort study, 36% of patients who had experienced a TIA developed a stroke during the next 10 years, with the greatest risk in the first 2 months. Over 50% of strokes occuring in a cohort of TIA patients occur within 1 year of the first ischaemic episode.

Case–control studies have demonstrated that the use of oral contraceptives increases the incidence of strokes. The use of exogenous oestrogens in men (e.g. high doses of stilboestrol in the treatment of prostatic cancer) increases the risk of stroke.

There is a strong negative correlation with vitamin C intake and some evidence to implicate the use of tobacco in the aetiology of cerebrovascular disease in men. Genetic predisposition to stroke appears to be weak.

Prevention

Treatment of hypertension has been shown to lower the incidence of stroke. The risk is reduced at all levels of blood pressure but especially in individuals with markedly elevated pressures. The beneficial effect of lowering blood pressure is well proven for first strokes and there is evidence (although from smaller studies) that it also holds for later episodes. There is no evidence that treatment of diabetes results in a reduction of stroke risk.

VARICOSE VEINS

These are dilatations of the superficial veins of the lower limb, resulting from faulty valves in saphenous veins and in the perforating veins which connect the superficial and deep venous systems.

Epidemiology

Varicose veins do not threaten life and are seldom disabling, but they cause a considerable demand for medical care. The prevalence of varicose veins varies markedly and is highest in developed countries. During one year in the USA 1% of the population sees a doctor at least once because of varicose veins and almost 100 000 excision and ligation operations are carried out, each causing an average stay of 6.4 days in hospital. Studies in Israel and Michigan have shown a prevalence among women aged 20 and over of around 1 in 3. The female:male ratio is between 2 and 3.

Varicose veins are positively associated with weight; several studies have shown an association with prolonged standing and with habitual corset wearing. There is little epidemiological evidence for an association with parity (when the effect of age is controlled). Dietary causes, especially a low intake of fibre, have been suggested. The possible mechanisms include pressure by the loaded bowel on the external iliac veins and transmission of pressure to the leg veins as a result of a need to strain at stool. Other speculative causes include the use of raised toilets rather than squatting at stool and the effect on the saphenous vein of sitting on chairs rather than the ground during childhood.

Prevention

It appears likely that varicose veins can be partly prevented by avoiding obesity, abstaining from habitual prolonged standing and avoiding the use of tight foundation garments. A high fibre diet may also help to prevent the condition.

6

Diseases of the respiratory system

CHRONIC BRONCHITIS

For the epidemiologist, the diagnosis of chronic bronchitis rests on symptoms rather than physical signs. Many epidemiological studies have used the questionnaire devised by the Medical Research Council, or others similar to it. Using such questionnaires, the formulation of symptomatic definitions has been possible and one such is: 'chronic or recurrent cough with expectoration on most days for at least 3 months in the year during at least 2 consecutive years'. It is now recognized that what used to be regarded as a single disease comprises at least two distinct pathological processes:

1. A hypersecretory disorder characterized by expectoration with increasing liability to clinical bronchial infections.
2. An obstructive disorder characterized by intrinsic airways disease with or without emphysema, causing eventual disability.

Epidemiology

Chronic bronchitis has been a major cause of fatal illness in Europe for at least two centuries and nowadays affects all industrialized countries. Large differences in respiratory mortality occur between countries but it is not known how much the reported rates reflect variations in diagnostic practices. However, there is little doubt that in Britain chronic bronchitis is an important health problem. It is the largest single cause of loss of work and, because of its high prevalence, has been termed 'the English disease'.

The great London smog of December 1952 gave a tremendous stimulus to research into chronic bronchitis: 4000 excess cardiorespiratory deaths occurred within a week, mainly in middle-aged and elderly people already suffering from chronic cardiovascular or respiratory diseases, and hospital wards were filled with bronchitic patients who had been suddenly precipitated into cardiorespiratory failure.

In a national survey conducted by the Royal College of General Practitioners in 1961–62, the prevalence in the age group 40–64 years was 17% in men and 8% in women. It represents 14% of all deaths from non-violent causes. The male/female ratio of deaths is 3:1.

The mortality rate is twice as high in cities compared with rural areas. Chronic bronchitis prevalence and mortality are both higher in areas of high atmospheric pollution and in dusty occupations (e.g. coal-miners, standardized mortality ratio (SMR) 200; foundary workers, SMR 150). In Britain mortality is highest in the heavily industrialized areas in Scotland and the north of England. These regional differences are principally in the obstructive type of chronic bronchitis.

There is a steep social class gradient in prevalence and mortality both in men and in women; in each social class, rates are highest in men. The prevalence of chronic bronchitis increases with age. Both in the UK and the USA bronchitis mortality is higher in the winter than the summer. In England and Wales since the early 1950s there has been a marked decrease in bronchitis mortality in women at all ages, but in men only below 65 years.

At all ages, the prevalence of chronic bronchitis is greater in smokers than in non-smokers, and smoking is now a more important aetiological factor than air pollution (*Fig. 6.1*). In non-smokers, air pollution has little effect on the prevalence of chronic bronchitis whereas in smokers the effect is very much greater. Both types of chronic bronchitis are caused predominantly by smoking (particularly of cigarettes) and develop in people with constitutional susceptibility, the nature of which is not known. The forced expiratory

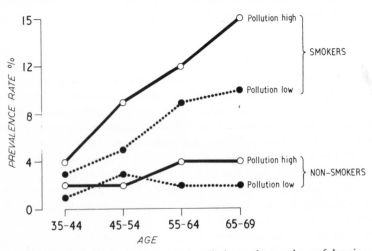

Fig. 6.1 The effect of smoking and of atmospheric pollution on the prevalence of chronic bronchitis. (Source: Lambert & Reid 1970 Lancet 1: 853–857.)

volume declines with age, but it declines more rapidly in smokers than in non-smokers.

Mortality from chronic bronchitis increases progressively with the number of cigarettes smoked. In men who smoke 25 or more cigarettes a day, the death rate from the disease (or from emphysema) is over 20 times greater than in non-smokers of the same age and sex, and among all cigarette smokers it is 12 times greater. Mortality from chronic bronchitis among male doctors who had given up smoking for more than 5 years was shown by Doll and Hill to be only a quarter of that in those who continued to smoke or had given up for less than 5 years.

In childhood, the incidence of lower respiratory tract infections is related to levels of air pollution but there is no such relationship in upper respiratory tract infections. Cough and phlegm are more common in children who smoke — and in the children of parents who smoke. People who develop severe chronic bronchitis in middle life have had more sickness absence due to re-spiratory causes in the early years of working life than have matched controls. It has also been shown that respiratory symptoms in early adult life are often related to lower respiratory tract disease in early childhood.

Prevention

The most important preventive measure is undoubtedly the exhorting of smokers to give up the practice and encouraging young people not to start. The hypersecretory type of chronic bronchitis usually remits when smoking ceases; in the obstructive type, the decline in forced expiratory volume is slowed down. A group worthy of special attention in these health education measures are smokers who already have a forced expiratory volume signif-icantly below the population average for their sex, age and height. Another clinical measure of importance is the adequate treatment of lower respiratory tract infection in children.

It is likely that particulate pollution of the air is of greater importance in the aetiology of chronic bronchitis than gaseous pollution, e.g. by sulphur dioxide. Considerable progress has been made in recent decades (through the application of the Clean Air Act) in reducing levels of particulate pollution and these measures need to be continued and extended further.

PNEUMOCONIOSIS

The pneumoconioses are lung diseases caused by the inhalation of dust. Those due to mineral dusts include silicosis, asbestosis and coalworkers' pneumoconiosis. Those due to organic (vegetable) dusts include byssinosis (cotton, flax, hemp), bagassosis (sugarcane pulp) and farmers' lung (spores growing in mouldy hay).

Epidemiology

The inhalation of dust in the working environment has long been known to cause lung diseases. Hippocrates described the metal digger as a man who breathes with difficulty and Agricola observed in 1556 that the dust in the mines of the Carpathian Mountains 'penetrates into the lungs and produces difficulty in breathing. . . women are found who have married seven husbands, all of whom this terrible consumption has carried off to a premature death.'

The pneumoconioses are among the 'Prescribed Diseases' entitling affected workers to financial compensation from the State. Despite the attendant investigative and notification procedures, these data give only an approximate guide to incidence and prevalence rates; they can be obtained with accuracy only by means of careful field studies. Most pneumoconioses are chronic conditions that present insidiously with dyspnoea on exertion. Because of this insidious onset, early ascertainment of cases is difficult. Most investigations of incidence and prevalence rely on regular screening using standardized methods for clinical evaluation (such as the Medical Research Council questionnaire on respiratory symptoms), assessment of radiological abnormality (such as the standard films issued by the International Labour Organization) and respiratory function.

Coalworkers' pneumoconsis is by far the most common form of industrial lung disease but the prevalence has been falling for several decades. It is high in South Wales because of anthracite mining. Simple pneumoconiosis, in which there is little tissue reaction, appears earliest in those exposed to the highest dust concentration; it is therefore more common in coalface workers than those employed elsewhere in the mines. Complicated pneumoconiosis (characterized by local masses of dense fibrosis heavily loaded with dust) rarely develops in those with minor degrees of simple pneumoconiosis.

The prevalence of coalworkers' pneumoconiosis varies in UK collieries from 5 to 60% and depends on the dust levels, the physical and chemical properties of the dust, the age distribution of the miners, the labour turnover and the proportion of coalface workers.

Complicated pneumoconiosis, especially in older men when the disease is in the more advanced stages, can lead to severe disability. Mortality is little increased in simple pneumoconiosis; in complicated pneumoconiosis mortality depends upon the severity of the condition. The presence of silica in the lung predisposes to tuberculosis and at autopsy 40% of cases of complicated pneumoconiosis have evidence of tuberculosis.

The significant epidemiological findings in other pneumoconioses are: the severity of symptoms in byssinosis after a period away from work, e.g. on return to work on Monday mornings; a high prevalence of byssinosis in those most exposed to the dust, e.g. card room workers in whom the prevalence may reach 50%; and the acute respiratory symptoms of farmers' lung following exposure to mouldy hay.

Prevention

The pneumoconioses are preventable provided the inhalation of respirable particles over a working lifetime is kept below the level required to give rise to the disease. Guidelines for 'threshold limit values' are published and these are modified as new data become available. Dust prevention in industry is expensive but not insuperable; the standards which have been set are within the competence of industrial engineers.

ASTHMA

Asthma is characterized by periodic attacks of breathlessness caused by obstruction of the airways which is variable in degree and largely reversible, either spontaneously or as a result of treatment. It may occur in acute attacks, with free intervals lasting from hours to days or even years, or it may occur as a chronic state in which the patient has frequent minor and major exacerbations of the disease.

Epidemiology

The Second National Survey of Morbidity in General Practice indicated that approximately 500 000 individuals in England and Wales consulted a doctor at least once for asthma in 1970–71. It is likely that there are a million asthmatics in Britain, many of whom do not consult their doctor because their symptoms are mild. Up to the age of 15 years, 2–3% of boys have asthma and about 1–2% of girls. The prevalence in adults is usually said to be 1–2%, but estimates vary widely because of the varying definitions of asthma.

Although asthma appears to be more common in children from better-off families, there is evidence that the prevalence of *severe* asthma is greatest in children of social class IV and V families.

The prognosis is worst if the asthma develops in the first 2 years of life. The more severe the disease, the more likely it is to continue into adult life. A follow-up study of children with asthma examined between 1948 and 1952 showed that 20 years later only 50% were symptom free. The most important adverse factors affecting prognosis are a family history of allergy and the existence of another atopic condition in the child, such as eczema.

Case fatality varies between 1 and 4%. Between 1960 and 1965 there was an eight-fold increase in the death rate from asthma among children aged 10–14 years in Britain, possibly due to greater use of pressurized bronchodilator aerosols containing sympathomimetic amines.

A family history of asthma or other manifestations of hypersensitivity are present in half to three-quarters of cases. The nature of genetic factors and mode of inheritance are unknown. The presence of disease in the mother has much greater significance than disease in the father. A child with asthma is twice as likely to have an affected mother as an affected father. There is a postive family history of asthma in about 60% of cases, hay fever in 30% and atopic dermatitis in about 20%. The concordance rate in monozygotic twins is 25% and in dizygotic twins 16%.

The allergens that are of importance in asthma are pollens, moulds, bacteria and foods such as cows' milk and egg proteins. Sensitivity to house dust is relatively common and many believe that the house dust mite plays a large part in causing asthma attacks. The mite lives in a warm damp environment and its main food appears to be shed skin scales. These accumulate in bedding and may account for some children having asthma attacks in the early hours of the morning. A child with one form of atopic disease, whether it be hay fever, dermatitis, rhinitis or asthma, will often subsequently develop another atopic disorder.

The onset of asthma is often associated with an acute respiratory tract infection. It is not known whether allergic children get more viral infections than the non-allergic. Children with asthma are often more emotionally disturbed and more intelligent than control children, but educational attainments are not greater. Some attacks of asthma are precipitated by psychological factors. In one study emotional states such as fear, excitement or anger were responsible for about 35% of attacks of asthma. Environmental factors (such as humidity or cold) may be important in the exacerbation of asthma.

Prevention

Hyposensitization, protection against allergens, hypnosis and psychotherapy all have a place in preventing asthmatic attacks. The best results with hyposensitization occur in children suffering from pollen-determined seasonal asthma and hay fever. Mite-sensitive children can often be helped by measures directed at reducing the mite population (e.g. vacuum cleaning all rooms at least twice weekly, using only bedding made of synthetic materials, changing sheets and pillow cases weekly, airing the bedding in direct sunlight) and keeping pets (which should be washed with a special shampoo periodically) outdoors if possible. The best results from hypnosis and psychotherapy are in children who are overanxious and insecure.

CARCINOMA OF THE LARYNX

There are two types — intrinsic carcinoma arising from the interior of the larynx, usually from the anterior half of one of the vocal cords, and extrinsic carcinoma which attacks the epiglottis, aryepiglottic fold or posterior surface of the cricoid cartilage.

Epidemiology

The highest incidences have been found in India and South American countries. Laryngeal cancer is most common in Caucasians and in urban dwellers. It represents 1.5–2% of all malignancies in the UK where there are 1800 new cases each year, 80% being men. The disease has become increasingly common in women since 1950 but there has been no such increase in men. Case fatality is about 40%.

Very few cases occur before the age of 50 years but the incidence then increases up to 75 years. The SMR is three times greater in social class V than in social class I for males ages 15–64, but the difference is only twofold at later ages.

The most important risk factor is cigarette smoking, the incidence of laryngeal cancer rising linearly with the use of tobacco. Pipe and cigar smoking also confer a risk of the order of ten-fold over non-smokers. Occupational exposure to asbestos, nickel and wood dust constitute risk factors, especially in smokers. Alcohol consumption, especially excessive drinking, appears to increase the risk.

Prevention

There is good evidence that cessation of smoking reduces the risk of laryngeal cancer. Secondary prevention through the early investigation of hoarseness, arising 'out of the blue' and lasting more than 2 weeks, is advocated.

CARCINOMA OF THE BRONCHUS

Squamous cell tumours are the most common, accounting for more than half of all bronchial carcinoma. Undifferentiated growths account for nearly 40% of the total and adenocarcinoma for less than 10%.

Epidemiology

Neoplasms of the respiratory tract are of great importance because of their frequency and high mortality and because of the implication of environmental factors in their aetiology. Carcinoma of the bronchus has a bad prognosis which has been little altered by treatment with surgery, radiotherapy or chemotherapy. Overall survival at 5 years is less than 7%. The relatively short clinical course and lethal nature of bronchial carcinoma make it likely that mortality data provide a good approximation to the incidence of the disease. Bronchial carcinoma accounts for almost 9% of all deaths in men and 3% in women; it is responsible for more than a quarter of all cancer deaths in the UK.

About 5% of all cases of carcinoma of the bronchus are first discovered in asymptomatic persons on routine chest radiography.

The number of deaths from bronchial carcinoma continues to rise annually for both sexes although the rate of increase in women is much greater than for men. Age-specific death rates are falling in men under 75, although still rising in women over the age of 50. It has been postulated that bronchial carcinoma has always been a common disease but that in the past it was misdiagnosed. The accuracy of diagnosis has certainly improved, but this is unlikely to have played a significant part in the steep rise in mortality ascribed to bronchial carcinoma.

Tobacco smoking was first suggested as the cause of lung cancer in the 1920s and later atmospheric pollution and occupational exposures were implicated. It has been estimated that occupational exposures account for not more than 15% of lung cancer deaths. More than 50 retrospective studies and at least nine major prospective studies in several countries have shown an association between tobacco smoking and the the subsequent development of lung cancer.

In 1950 Doll and Hill published a preliminary report on their case–control study of smoking and carcinoma of the bronchus. Hospital patients with lung cancer were asked about their smoking habits and were compared with a non-cancer control group of general hospital patients, matched for sex and age. The study showed not only a great excess of smokers in the lung cancer group but also evidence of the dose–response relationship. Subsequent studies amply confirmed these findings, expanding the observations on dose to include not only the number of cigarettes smoked but also ways of smoking (inhalation) and the tar content of cigarette smoke. Those starting to smoke early in life were found to have a much higher risk. These studies have also shown an increased lung cancer risk associated with cigar and pipe smoking, but substantially less than that associated with cigarettes.

A causal association with cigarette smoking can explain the remarkable trend in lung cancer mortality in Britain and other countries during this century. Cigarette smoking amongst men increased in popularity towards the end of the last century but women only took up the habit during the First, and to a much greater extent the Second, World War. Since then there have been downward trends for smoking in men, with a more consistent decrease in men in younger age groups, but in women the steady upward trend has continued. The decline in mortality from lung cancer in younger men in recent years can be attributed not only to less smoking, but also to the increasing use of filter tipped cigarettes and of cigarettes with a lower tar content.

A 20-year prospective study on male British doctors by Doll and Hill lends

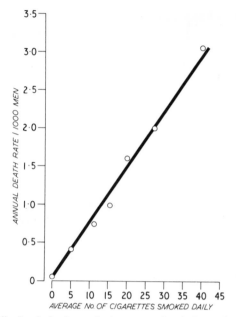

Fig. 6.2 Age-standardized male death rates for lung cancer in relation to cigarette smoking.

further evidence of a causal association between cigarette smoking and lung cancer (*Fig. 6.2*). The distinctive features of this study were the completeness of follow-up and the accuracy of death certification. Doctors reduced their cigarette consumption over the years of the study and lung cancer death rates in doctors have progressively declined and are now far below the national rates. Mortality from other cancers has not changed in the same way. This and other studies have shown that the relative reduction in risk becomes apparent within a few years of stopping smoking and that after about 10 years' abstention the ex-smokers' risk approached that of non-smokers (*Fig. 6.3*).

Confirmatory evidence for a causal association is provided by the finding of pre-malignant changes in the bronchial epithelium of smokers who have died of other diseases, with a decrease in frequency after giving up smoking, and by animal experiments which demonstrate that many carcinogenic substances are present in cigarette smoke. A genetic hypothesis has been postulated for the association between smoking and lung cancer but this does not fit the evidence, in particular with regard to the temporal changes in lung cancer mortality and the different mortality rates between the sexes.

Mortality rates are highest in large conurbations and it is believed the differences in smoking habits between town and country dwellers could account for part of the difference. Specific occupational exposures cannot account for

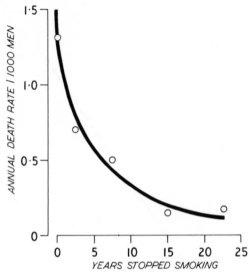

Fig. 6.3 Age-standardized male death rates for lung cancer in relation to the length of time they had given up smoking.

the consistently higher mortality from lung cancer in urban than in rural areas. While atmospheric pollution may be in part responsible for the greater lung cancer mortality in urban areas, even where differences in smoking habits are taken into account, the data suggest the presence of an additional urban factor.

Prevention

Strategies for the prevention of lung cancer caused by smoking are based on (1) the education of the public on the harmful effects of smoking and attempts to discourage smoking, especially by children; (2) limitation of cigarette advertising; and (3) attempts to produce a less harmful cigarette. If the effect of these measures is judged by the pattern of cigarette consumption, then they have so far been inadequate except perhaps for the reduction in smoking seen in persons in social class I.

MESOTHELIOMA

This is a histological description of a specific neoplasm of the pleura or peritoneum, the great majority of cases being pleural. All cases prove fatal.

Epidemiology

This disease — of which there are less than 150 cases each year in the UK — has gained importance because of its association with asbestos exposure. Its epidemiology is determined mainly by the history and distribution of asbestos mining and use; thus the incidence of mesothelioma is highest in countries such as Canada, South Africa and the USSR where it is mined. It is relatively common in asbestos workers, especially pipe laggers and former shipyard workers. The current increase in incidence is a consequence of the rise in battleship building during the Second World War, the latent period being usually 30–40 years. As dust control measures did not improve until the late 1960s, it is probable that no reduction in the incidence of mesothelioma will occur during this century.

The small-fibre blue asbestos (crocidolite) appears to be the most damaging agent. It is likely that cigarette smoking exacerbates the risk. The excess of cases in men and the peak incidence at age 70 are related to occupational exposure, a history of which is obtained in up to 90% of cases. The higher rates in manual, especially skilled, workers is also a function of occupational exposure. Mesothelioma may arise after a relatively low dose of inhaled asbestos. Industries involving sufficient exposure include textile and brake manufacturing, building, shipbuilding and repairing, and marine engineering. Removal of old lagging is particularly hazardous. The occurrence of the disease following household exposure (through handling dusty working clothes) is well authenticated.

Prevention

The association between asbestos and mesothelioma represents an example of how epidemiological associations can influence society. Asbestos is indispensable to many branches of modern industrial technology and the production of crocidolite is currently increasing at a greater rate than other forms of asbestos. With the additional hazard of asbestosis and bronchial carcinoma there is now strict control over the use of asbestos and of dust levels while the search for alternative materials develops. Because of the very long latent period, the effect of these measures will not be realized in a reduced incidence for many years.

Diseases of the digestive system

DENTAL DISEASES

The principal conditions are dental caries and periodontal disease. The former is a disease in which there is destruction of the tooth substance, and the latter is one in which the attachment of the tooth to the alveolar bone is progressively destroyed. These two diseases constitute the main reasons for tooth loss.

Epidemiology

Reliable statistics are lacking for many countries, but there is good evidence that the incidence of caries is substantially less in developing countries than in the developed world. The highest recorded rates are in Scandinavia and New Zealand. Within the UK, the incidence is highest in Scotland, Wales, Devon and Cornwall.

Caries incidence has been shown in several countries to be inversely related to the concentration of the fluoride in drinking water (*Fig. 7.1*). In the low fluoride areas where fluoride has been added to bring the level to 1 part per million, the incidence of caries has fallen. A well-known example is the 50% reduction that occurred in Kilmarnock when fluoride was added between 1956 and 1961. A decision in 1961 to cease the fluoridation led to an increase in caries incidence to its original level.

Dental caries is a disease of the early part of life. National surveys of dental health have shown that caries is present in two-thirds of children at the age of 5 years. It may begin as early as 2 years of age, and it continues to occur by separate individual attacks on specific anatomical sites in a sequential order. This process continues up to about 40 years but very few, if any, fresh teeth succumb beyond this age. The ceiling level of attack averages 24 teeth per person — seven deciduous and 17 permanent teeth. It is an important feature of dental caries that a substantial proportion of teeth never succumb and that a small percentage of people can remain caries-free throughout life. Of the 24 teeth currently likely to succumb, 50% do so by 12 years of age, 70% by 15

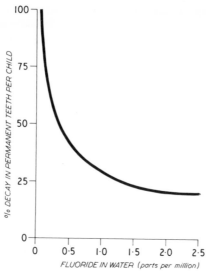

Fig. 7.1 Dental decay in children: the relationship with the fluorine content of water.

years and 80% by 25 years. In a fluoridated community the average ceiling level of attacked teeth is reduced by 10.

Since about 1960, there has been a decrease in the incidence of dental caries in both fluoride and non-fluoride communities, particularly up to age 5 years. The mean number of attacked teeth by age 5 years has fallen from about 5 to 2.5. In fluoride communities this figure has fallen from about 2.5 to 1.2. As yet we do not know if, and to what extent, this fall has extended into adulthood. The reason for this fall, which seems widespread in most industrialized countries, is not known with certainty; the most likely reason is the use of fluoride toothpaste. In Japan, where its use is almost unknown, caries incidence has not changed. In countries where there is widespread fluoridation of water (in Britain only about 10% drink fluoridated water), this has probably played a large part. In developing countries caries is increasing, presumably due to an increased sugar intake.

In twin studies there is a higher concordance rate in identical twins than in non-identical twins in childhood; similar studies are now being conducted in young adults.

There are several kinds of periodontal disease but that with the greatest prevalence and the most serious clinical consequences is the chronic condition in which there is progressive loss of the fibres which attach the tooth to the alveolar bone. The natural history of this condition is very different from that of dental caries; it is confined to permanent teeth and in Britain it does not become clinically manifest much before 25 years of age. All persons in all countries and all teeth are at risk and gradually succumb as age advances.

Treatment has not been very successful and periodontal disease is a major reason for total tooth loss after 25 years of age. Fluorides in drinking water do not reduce the incidence of the progressive loss of attachment of the tooth to alveolar bone.

Edentulousness (total tooth loss) before 25 years is nearly always a consequence of dental caries; at that age about 6% of British people have lost all their teeth as a consequence of this disease. At the present time in England about 25% are edentulous by 40 years of age, 50% by 50 years, 75% by 60 years, and 80% by 70 years. In Scotland and in the North of England these levels are achieved about 5 years earlier.

Prevention

Fluoridation of water supplies to a level of 1 part per million together with the use of fissure sealants can reduce the incidence of caries by at least 75%. While other methods of administering fluoride (such as topical fluoride applications and toothpastes) may delay the onset of disease, there is no evidence of long-term benefit. To date dietary changes seem to have had little value as preventive measures.

ORAL CANCER

Cancer of the lip, tongue, oropharnyx and hypopharnyx are included under this heading. Most of these neoplasms are squamous cell carcinomas. Case-fatality rates vary from 15% for lip to 70% for pharynx.

Epidemiology

Of these tumours, cancer of the lip is the one that is subject to most variation in incidence; it is especially common in rural dwellers and fishermen, presumably reflecting the effect of exposure to sunlight. Oral cancer is most prevalent in India and South East Asia.

Most of these cancers are more common in the lower social classes. Cancer of the tongue is also common in social class I and it is possible that pipe-smoking contributes to its pathogenesis. In India cancer of the tongue probably accounts for 20% of all malignancies. Wide international variations are being explained by betel-nut chewing, and the use of tobacco (smoking and chewing), all of which appear to be risk factors.

In most Western countries there has been a marked decline in the frequency of tongue carcinoma in men over the last 40 years. This is attributed to a decrease in smoking and tobacco chewing and also to improved oral hygiene. However, during the same period the incidence has increased in women, probably reflecting a greater prevalence of smoking.

Chronic excessive alchohol intake is a risk factor, possibly acting through the associated dietary deficiencies or by facilitating the local absorption and potency of carcinogens, such as tobacco, in the mouth.

There is a relatively higher frequency of cancer of the tongue in heavy pipe and cigar smokers. The risk of developing a squamous cell carcincoma at any site in the oral cavity is 15 times greater in alcohol-drinking smokers than it is in non-drinking smokers.

Syphilis is a risk factor but it is not known whether it is a primary factor or whether syphilis patients are most susceptible to oral cancer as a result of other behavioural and socioeconomic factors.

Prevention

A reduction in smoking, alcohol intake and betel-nut chewing are the preventive measures likely to bring about a fall in the incidence of these malignancies.

CANCER OF THE SALIVARY GLANDS

The parotid is the gland most often affected; 75% of salivary gland tumours are plemorphic adenomas and 15% carcinomas.

Epidemiology

The highest incidences are found in Eskimos, in Chinese and in Hawaii. There are about 500 new cases each year in the UK but the incidence is declining by 2% per annum. The incidence increases with age although cases do occur in young people. Up to the age of 55, the disease is more common in women, thereafter in men. Rural dwellers seem to be at greater risk but there is no striking social class difference.

There are few clues to the causes of salivary gland cancer other than an excess in those exposed to radiation and an association with breast cancer.

Prevention

Little progress has been made in primary prevention. The policy of regarding all parotid neoplasms as potentially malignant may contribute to the relatively good prognosis.

CANCER OF THE OESOPHAGUS

These are mostly squamous cell carcinomas except those (about 5%) arising in ectopic gastric mucosa at the lower end of the oesophagus. The majority of the neoplasms occur in the lower third of the oesophagus. Most cases prove fatal.

Epidemiology

The incidence is exceptionally high in certain parts of the world including the Iranian and Russian borders of the Caspian Sea, Northern China, Transkei and Zimbabwe (in blacks). The disease is more common in Northern France (Normandy and Brittany) than in the rest of Europe. In the USA, the incidence is doubled in the black population.

In the UK, mortality from oesophageal cancer fell by 50% between 1930 and 1960 but in recent years has risen again; registrations have increased by 2% per annum during the past decade. There are almost 4000 cases each year in the UK.

The incidence increases sharply with age and is almost twice as great in men as in women. In many countries, oesophageal cancer is more common in urban dwellers.

Under 65 years the disease appears to be less common in non-manual occupations (SMR 83) and most common in the unskilled (SMR 139). However, in the elderly, the class mortality curve is U-shaped with the highest mortality in social classes I and V.

Although a number of risk factors have been identified, the marked international variation has not been explained other than by vague dietary imbalances and poverty. The high incidence in some parts of Africa has been attributed to the consumption of beer made from maize. In developed countries, where the incidence is less high, the major risk factors are cigarette smoking (which increases the risk by a factor of at least two) and alcohol (which is responsible for the excess incidence in Northern France). In the UK the cohort of men born about 1906 has had a lower incidence than other cohorts. This correlates closely with alcohol consumption during early adult life.

Prevention

In Western countries, alcohol and smoking represent avoidable hazards. In the regions of China where the incidence is high, screening by brush biopsy has been introduced to enable early diagnosis.

PEPTIC ULCER

This is a breach in the mucosa of the stomach or duodenum. When chronic, it is associated with surrounding fibrosis and subsequent scarring. Acute ulcers are not considered here.

Epidemiology

Gastric and duodenal ulcers are both common conditions in Europe, with duodenal ulcer being consistently two to three times more common. However, during the nineteenth century, gastric ulcer was the predominant lesion in Britain and it was mainly a disease of young women. The prevalence of duodenal ulcer began to increase at the beginning of the present century and, for the last 50 years, it has been more common than gastric ulcer in most areas. The prevalence of duodenal ulcer may have reached a peak in the mid-1950s and may now be declining, albeit slowly. A striking fall has occurred in peptic ulcer perforation rates in men and bleeding has replaced perforation as the main complication.

Mortality and hospital admission rates for gastric and duodenal ulcer have fallen in the last 20 years in England and Wales. This fall has been more obvious in men than in women and has been particularly pronounced for duodenal ulcer in recent years. The prevalence of peptic ulcer, particularly duodenal ulcer, seems to have fallen, but the extent of the reduction is difficult to determine. Possible reasons for the fall are: more accurate diagnosis, new drug treatments for dyspepsia and the frequent use of gastrectomy in the 1950s and 1960s. Hospital discharge statistics suggest that, within Britain, duodenal ulcer is more common in the north than in the south, but that there is no consistent variation in gastric ulcer.

Incidence and prevalence rates are difficult to obtain and published statistics are based mainly on hospital discharges, death registrations and autopsy surveys. In Western Europe the mean annual incidence per 1000 aged 15 and over is approximately: gastric ulcer — men 0.5, women 0.3; duodenal ulcer — men 2.2, women 0.6. Prevalence rates are much higher. 10% or more of Western populations may be affected at some time in their lives. Peptic ulcer accounts for approximately 10% of all adult admissions to general hospitals.

A high prevalence of duodenal ulcer compared with gastric ulcer has also been reported from North America and Australia. Gastric ulcer appears to be less common in the USA and Canada than it is in Britain. Studies in several African countries and in India have shown that almost all ulcers are duodenal and that they almost all occur in men. They tend to give rise to pyloric obstruction, with bleeding and perforation being relatively uncommon.

Gastric ulcer deaths have been consistently more frequent in those of unskilled occupations and duodenal ulcer deaths now show a similar pattern. These social class differences may be partly explained by differences in the quality of medical care obtained. Gastric ulcer incidence rises after the age of 40. Duodenal ulcer is rare before the age of 20 but the incidence then rises progressively.

Both the prevalence and mortality rates for peptic ulcer are higher in smokers than in non-smokers. Both types of ulcer have a raised incidence in persons of blood group O and in non-secretors. There is an association between peptic ulcer and coffee intake, with an apparently protective effect of milk, but these associations are not necessarily causal.

Prevention

It is likely that secular changes in duodenal ulcer prevalence are related to diet, but its aetiological significance is still unknown. Education about the harmful effect of smoking is at present the only method of primary prevention.

CANCER OF THE STOMACH

Most of these tumours are adenocarcinomas. At least 90% of cases prove fatal.

Epidemiology

Gastric cancer is particularly common in Japan, Chile, Colombia, Finland and parts of the USSR. It is the second most common cause of cancer death in men in the UK (after bronchus) and ranks fourth in women (breast, bronchus and colon being the leading sites). There are over 12 000 registrations annually in England alone, 60% of cases occurring in the age range 65–79 years. The incidence increases with age; it is more common in males at all ages, and by a factor of 2.5 in the age range 40–74 years.

There is a very marked social class gradient, the SMR in social class V being three times that in class I. This probably explains the higher rates in urban areas and in the North of England and in Wales. There has been a reduction in incidence in all Western countries during the last 50 years, the fall having been greatest in women. Nevertheless, gastric cancer is still responsible for 2% of all deaths and 10% of cancer deaths in the UK.

The incidence in migrants changes over two or more generations. Studies of migrants from Japan (where the incidence of gastric cancer is high) to the USA (where the incidence is much lower) suggest that diet is an important factor.

A number of risk factors have been identified, most of which are consistent with the hypothesis that dietary nitrate, converted to nitrite by bacterial action, leads to the production of carcinogenic nitrosamines.

1. The incidence is high in areas where there are rich nitrate deposits in the soil, either occurring naturally or due to their use as a fertilizer. This may explain the high incidence in South American countries. An association with the nitrate content of drinking water has also been demonstrated.

2. The chemical preservation of food (such as pickling and curing) involves the use of nitrates. This helps to explain the high incidence of gastric cancer in Japan. The recent decline in incidence in 'Westernized' countries is at least partly explained by the use of refrigeration rather than chemical methods in the preservation of food.
3. Case–control studies have suggested that the consumption of fresh vegetables and milk may protect against gastric cancer. It is probable that vitamin C and other characteristics of these foods inhibit the conversion of nitrites to nitrosamines, or of nitrates to nitrites.
4. There is a four-fold increase in the risk of gastric cancer in achlorhydric conditions such as atrophic gastritis, pernicious anaemia and following partial gastrectomy for duodenal ulcer. The absence of acid encourages the production of nitrites, and thus nitrosamines, from ingested nitrate. The recently introduced histamine-2 blockers which inhibit the release of gastric acid may, in long-term use, represent a similar risk.

A number of other risk factors have also been suggested:

1. Cigarette smoking increases the risk, particularly of carcinoma of the cardia.
2. An association with red wine consumption in France has been demonstrated by a case–control study and by regional statistics.
3. Gastric cancer is more common in coal miners and workers in the metal and rubber industries.
4. It has long been believed that gastric ulcer is a pre-malignant condition. Cancer is sometimes observed to arise in a pre-existing ulcer and there is an association with gastric ulcer in national incidence data. However, this association disappears when regional data are analysed and a longitudinal study in Sweden has shown no increased risk in ulcer patients.

Prevention

As has been mentioned, the replacement of chemical preservation of food by refrigeration has almost certainly been important in reducing the incidence of gastric cancer. To cease using nitrate fertilisers is impracticable at present.

Care should be taken in the long-term use of drugs that inhibit gastric acid secretion.

In Japan, where gastric cancer affects 10% of men, attempts have been made to diagnose the disease at an early and curable stage. When the lesion is confined to the submucosa, cure rates up to 90% have been reported. Where the disease is common, screening of middle-aged men is cost-effective. In the UK, USA and other countries where the incidence is lower, screening by endoscopy and cytology of gastric juice would prove very costly. It is accepted, however, that immediate access to such diagnostic facilities for new dyspeptic patients might help to reduce the duration between the first symptom and operation (currently an average of 7 months) and therefore improve the prognosis.

DIVERTICULAR DISEASE

Diverticular disease of the colon included both diverticulosis and diverticulitis. Diverticulosis is a common finding at barium enema and at autopsy in Western countries, but the clinical pattern associated with it is extremely variable; an unknown proportion has no symptoms. The commonest form of diverticular disease in Western countries is diverticulosis localized to the sigmoid colon.

Epidemiology

Although commonly detected in Western Europe, North America and Australia, diverticular disease of the sigmoid colon is uncommon in rural Africa and Asia. Crude death rates for diverticular disease have risen ten-fold in the past 50 years in England and Wales but this can be explained by the increasing sophistication of radiological techniques, changing patterns in death certification and the increasing proportion of the elderly in the population.

The disease appears in Africans and Asians who have either been reared in the West on a fibre-deficient diet or who have adopted Western eating habits. Bowel transit times seem on average to be shorter and stool weight to be greater in Africans living on traditional diets. In Britain the prevalence of diverticular disease increases with age and there appears to be no sex difference. Death due to diverticular disease is rare.

Prevention

An adequate intake of dietary fibre appears to be a reasonable preventive measure. It increases stool bulk, lowers the intraluminal pressure and decreases the transit time.

INFLAMMATORY BOWEL DISEASES

The two chronic disorders included under this term are ulcerative colitis and Crohn's disease. Ulcerative colitis is a diffuse mucosal inflammation which begins in the rectum and may affect the whole colon. Crohn's disease may affect any part of the gastrointestinal tract, but the ileocaecal region is the area most commonly involved.

Epidemiology

Both diseases occur worldwide, but are most common in Western countries. Studies in Britain and Sweden show that the incidence of Crohn's disease has been increasing, although the peak may now have been reached.

Ulcerative colitis predominantly affects young adults; patients with Crohn's disease are usually between 20 and 60 years of age at diagnosis. The incidence of ulcerative colitis is slightly higher in women than in men but the difference is not great.

There is no HLA association in either disease except for patients who also have sacro-ileitis, a quarter whom are HLA-B27 positive. Both diseases occur more commonly within families than would be expected by chance, but the basis for this familial incidence is not clear.

Prevention

The aetiology of these diseases is unknown and no preventive measures have been identified.

APPENDICITIS

The diagnosis of acute appendicitis is obvious when there are localized abdominal pain, fever and signs of peritoneal inflammation. However, lesser grades of inflammation, which may be associated with recurrent pain reminiscent of appendicitis, often make the diagnosis difficult.

Epidemiology

Operation statistics are the only reliable basis for epidemiological studies of appendicitis. Appendicectomy is the commonest emergency operation in Western Europe and North America. Appendicitis was an unrecognized condition until 1886 and it seems likely that the increase in incidence over the last 100 years has been due to the adoption of a low-residue diet. In recent decades, the frequency of acute appendicitis appears to have fallen in the UK and the USA; however, in England and Wales the decrease in hospital admissions for acute appendicitis has been accompanied by an increase in admissions with abdominal pain of uncertain cause. In some countries, large variations in appendicectomy rates have been related to the ability to pay and to the diagnostic skills of doctors.

Before 1940, appendicitis was rare in sub-Saharal Africa but it is now becoming much more common and this is believed to be due to the acquisition of Western dietary practices. During the Second World War appendicitis began to appear for the first time among African troops after they had been supplied with British army rations. Evidence is accumulating which suggests that appendicitis occurs frequently only in populations in which solid faecal particles are commonly present in the lumen of the appendix. This is probably due to excessive absorption of water from the gut in the absence of sufficient fibre to retain it. A fall in the frequency of appendicitis in Switzerland during the Second World War has been ascribed to the widespread adoption of a vegetarian diet.

The disease has its highest incidence between the ages of 5 and 25 years with equal proportions of each sex being affected. When National Service recruits were examined in the 1950s appendicectomy had been performed in nearly twice as many with a grammar or independent school education as in those with a lower level of education. This may reflect differing social pressures over the need for investigation and treatment of abdominal pain, rather than a true difference in the frequency of the disease.

Prevention

If it is true that dietary fibre is important in preventing appendicitis, then this affords one measure by which the incidence can be reduced.

CANCER OF THE COLON

Most malignant tumours of the colon are adenocarcinomas. One-third occur in the caecum or ascending colon, half in the descending and sigmoid colon and the remainder in the transverse colon.

Epidemiology

The highest incidence is found in the USA; most Western countries have a high incidence but the disease is uncommon in Japan, Africa, Asia and most of South America.

Cancer of the colon is one of the most common diseases in the Western world. In the UK, there are 15 000 new cases each year and almost 11 000 deaths. The 5 year survival rate is 30%. The incidence increases sharply with age and is marginally higher in women up to the age of 60 years, and higher in men by 5–10% in the elderly. The incidence in migrants changes very quickly — faster than for any cancer other than that of the skin.

Throughout the world, the incidence of colon cancer tends to be greater in the higher social classes, the difference being greatest in the less affluent countries; in the UK the excess mortality in social class I is confined to the elderly.

Although mortality has fallen by about 40% since 1940, this can be attributed to improved survival rates rather than a change in incidence. Indeed recent evidence suggests that the incidence of colon cancer is increasing slowly in developed countries, but even faster in countries which are becoming westernized.

Most of the international and class variations in colon cancer can be explained in terms of dietary differences, most hypotheses being concerned with beef, animal fat and fibre. A number of case–control studies have suggested that beef intake is a risk factor. A dose–response effect is seen only among low-risk populations and low-intake groups, suggesting a threshold phenomenon. This would explain the diminishing social class variation with increasing affluence. Fat intake is associated with beef; a plausible aetiology, through the release of bile acids and their conversion to carcinogens, has been proposed.

Consistent results in recent studies suggest that dietary fibre protects against colon cancer. In British studies, fibre pentose correlates more closely with regional cancer incidence than other components of fibre. It appears likely that both fibre and beef are intimately concerned with the aetiology of colon cancer, one protective and the other causal.

A number of pathological states increase the risk of colon cancer. The most important of these is familial polyposis, the prevalence of which is about 1 in 10 000. Inherited as an autosomal dominant (with 80% penetrance), it gives rise to malignant change by the age of 60 years in almost all those affected. Other colonic polyps also possess a risk of malignant change, especially those of more than 2 cm diameter. Ulcerative colitis is a further premalignant condition, especially when present for 10 years or more. The excess risk may be as great as ten-fold and neoplasms often arise in proximal parts of the colon unaffected by colitis. Interestingly, a history of cholecystectomy is often given by patients with proximal tumours.

Prevention

The prevention of colon cancer may be considered in three stages:

1. The avoidance of the major dietary risk factors — which is easier said than done. The inclusion of beef and the relative absence of fibre are part and parcel of the Western diet. However, it is unlikely than any major reduction in incidence will occur unless there is a major shift in dietary habits.
2. Prevention in those with premalignant conditions has been based on prophylactic colectomy. In the future, screening by colonoscopy may represent a conservative alternative.
3. The early detection of malignant disease is undoubtedly worthwhile from the point of view of survival. Sigmoidoscopic screening of healthy populations has met with poor compliance; in any case it can detect only the minority of neoplasms (those occurring in the sigmoid colon). Screening

of symptomatic populations by faecal occult blood testing is currently being evaluated.

CANCER OF THE RECTUM

Most of these neoplasms are adenocarcinomas and, in many ways, cancer of the rectum resembles colon cancer. However, there are sufficient epidemiological differences between the two diseases to consider rectal cancer as a distinct entity. About 10% of lesions occur at the recto-sigmoid junction, 2% in the anal canal and the remainder in the rectum itself.

Epidemiology

The geographical variation in rectal cancer is similar to that for the colon with the highest incidence being in developed countries. Denmark has the highest recorded incidence.

As with colon cancer, the incidence of rectal cancer is rising slowly, but mortality has fallen substantially owing to improved survival. There are almost 10 000 new cases of rectal cancer annually in the UK; two-thirds prove fatal. The incidence increases sharply with age up to 50 years, but less steeply thereafter. In younger subjects, rectal cancer is as common as colon cancer but is rather less common in the elderly. Unlike colon cancer, rectal cancer at all ages is more common in men than in women. Social class differences have not been noted.

The dietary risk factors mentioned for colon cancer have also been implicated in rectal cancer, but the associations are less close. In addition, alcohol consumption in the form of beer has been implicated in a number of case–control and time-trend studies.

Ulcerative colitis, Crohn's disease and rectal polyps are regarded as premalignant conditions. Pelvic irradiation for cervical or testicular cancer has also been identified as a risk factor.

Prevention

Dietary manipulation remains the best prospect for primary prevention. The ease with which the rectum can be examined allows the removal of polyps and regular visual screening for malignant change in other high risk groups. Screening of healthy and symptomatic populations is currently under evaluation.

HAEMORRHOIDS

They were at one time viewed as varicosities of the anal veins, but are now regarded as a prolapse of vascular submucosal anal cushions which, in their natural position and size, are normal structures encircling the anal canal.

Epidemiology

Since the diagnosis is imprecise and liable to include other anal conditions, it is difficult to estimate the prevalence of haemorrhoids. The prevalence appears to be very much lower in developing countries than in the developed world. This has been related to the fibre content of the diet. When it is low, as in Western countries, constipation is common; this leads to straining at stool which in turn engorges the submucosal anal cushion with rupturing of its attachments to the anal sphincters.

Haemorrhoidectomy rates have fallen substantially in Britain during the past decade. This may well reflect the increasing use of high-fibre foods, either lowering the incidence of the condition or conferring sufficient symptomatic relief to render hospital treatment unnecessary.

Prevention

The evidence suggests that a high-fibre diet has a protective effect.

CIRRHOSIS OF THE LIVER

Cirrhosis is a diffuse hepatic fibrosis which may result from a number of pathological processes. The less common types of cirrhosis (such as extrahepatic cholestasis, primary biliary cirrhosis, haemochromatosis, syphilitic cirrhosis) are not considered here.

Epidemiology

National mortality rates for cirrhosis correlate well with alcohol consumption and it is believed that between a half and two-thirds of cases in Britain are attributable to alcohol abuse. The risk of developing liver damage is related to the quantity drunk and the length of heavy drinking. People vary greatly in their susceptibility and women have a greater likelihood of liver damage than men.

Deaths from cirrhosis in Britain have increased by a quarter during the past decade. There has been a large increase recently in young men aged under 25. In men, the peak mortality is in the age group 50–60 years but the peak occurs about a decade earlier in women. Mortality in Britain is highest in social class I; in the USA it is highest in the lower socioeconomic group.

The highest risk is in occupations associated with the liquor trade or in which alcohol consumption is high.

Prevention

This lies in the control of alcohol abuse by changing the attitudes of society through health education and by fiscal measures.

CANCER OF THE LIVER

This includes primary liver cell carcinoma or hepatoma (90%) and intra-hepatic bile duct carcinoma or cholangiocarcinoma (10%). Both are almost always fatal.

Epidemiology

Cancer of the liver is an uncommon disease in most developed countries. There are less than 800 cases each year in the UK. The incidence is increasing slightly in developed countries. Hepatomata occur in the young, albeit rarely, but the incidence rises sharply with age up to 75 years, being at least twice as common in men. Hepatomata are extremely common in Central and South Africa (in blacks), South East Asia, Japan and Southern and Eastern Europe. In these high-risk areas, the incidence is high in young adults as well as in older people.

The major risk factor in developing countries is contamination of food with aflatoxin, a toxin produced by the fungus *Aspergillus flavus*. A dose–response effect of aflatoxin has been identified.

In developed countries, the main risk factors are cirrhosis of the liver (of all types) and chronic hepatitis-B virus infection. The geography of hepatoma in Europe follows closely that of the hepatitis-B virus carrier state. Cholangiocarcinoma is not associated with these risk factors; infection with *Chlonorchis sinensis* (a fluke) has been incriminated.

Prevention

Improved food preparation and preservation are the answer to the aflatoxin problem, but the rural, primitive nature of high-risk communities in the developing world makes this a distant target. The best hope for prevention in developed countries lies in immunization against hepatitis-B for those at increased risk of infection.

GALLSTONES

These contain varying proportions of bile pigments and cholesterol, together with other substances such as calcium and magnesium salts and bile acids.

Gallstones causing symptoms are probably outnumbered by asymptomatic stones.

Epidemiology

Epidemiological studies are hampered by the difficulties of determining the incidence and prevalence of the disease; asymptomatic stones are common, deaths are rare and autopsy data often do not represent the frequency in the total population. Although the number of cholecystectomies has increased steadily in recent decades, evidence from autopsy studies suggests that gall-stone frequency has not increased.

The prevalence of gallstones is high in Northern Europe and North America, and much lower in most tropical areas. They are 2–3 times more common in women than in men. The incidence and prevalence increase with age.

Standardized mortality ratios suggest a much greater prevalence of the disease in men of higher socioeconomic status; the reverse trend exists in wives.

Epidemiological support for an association between diet and gallstones is weak, but the one consistent feature is an association with obesity. There is also a negative association with ischaemic heart disease. There is no evidence that hereditary factors influence the incidence of gallstones.

Prevention

Dietary measures to prevent obesity may help to reduce the incidence of gallstones.

CANCER OF THE GALL-BLADDER AND BILIARY TRACT

These tumours are almost always adenocarcinomas: 50% occur in the gall-bladder itself, 35% in the extrahepatic bile duct and the remainder in the vicinity of the ampulla of Vater. Fatality is in excess of 95%.

Epidemiology

There are over 1000 cases each year in the UK. The incidence increases with age. There is a small excess in women but this is confined to gall-bladder neoplasms; bile duct tumours are slightly more common in men. There are no clear racial or social class variations.

Two clear-cut associations have been reported. One is the presence of gallstones which are 2–3 times more common in patients with gall-bladder cancer. However, it is not clear whether gallstones are an aetiological factor or the result of neoplasia, or whether the two diseases have a common cause. Secondly, infection and inflammation of the biliary tree represent well-defined risks. In New York, typhoid carriers with cholecystitis had a reported ten-fold increase in the risk of gall-bladder cancer. Similarly, a history of cholangitis is found more aften than expected in patients with bile duct cancer. The presumed mechanism is the conversion, by infection, of bile salts to carcinogens.

Prevention

The relationship between cholelithiasis and gall-bladder cancer is not clear but it has been proposed that dietary manipulation (reduction of fat and calorie intake) might reduce the incidence of both diseases. The prevalence of gall-bladder cancer in cholelithiasis is too low to justify screening for gall-stones in the absence of symptoms.

PANCREATITIS

Acute pancreatitis is characterized by abdominal pain and a grossly raised serum amylase. However, in chronic pancreatitis the diagnostic criteria are less clear and case ascertainment for epidemiological purposes is difficult.

Epidemiology

Pancreatitis is common in areas where the drinking of alcohol is customary. In Britain, deaths from acute pancreatitis have risen steadily in the past three decades, and this may be related to a rise in alcohol consumption. There is evidence from America that the incidence of pancreatitis (both acute and chronic) has risen.

Prevention

Education about the harmful effects of a high alcohol intake is the only present method of primary prevention.

CANCER OF THE PANCREAS

These common tumours are mostly adenocarcinoma; the disease is almost always fatal.

Epidemiology

The disease is most common in westernized countries; it is relatively uncommon in Eastern Europe, the Far East and Africa. The incidence in migrants changes rapidly, and black people living in Western countries have high rates.

Pancreatic cancer is responsible for almost 6000 deaths each year in the UK. The incidence has increased threefold since 1920. It is rare in the young, and the incidence increases sharply with age up to 75 years, being 50% more common in males at all ages. Under the age of 65 years there are no social class differences in mortality but in the elderly it is highest in class I.

The risk of pancreatic cancer is increased by a factor of two in smokers, diabetics and patients with a history of pancreatitis or gall-bladder disease. Workers in the chemical industry may be at increased risk.

Prevention

With the exception of smoking, no clearly preventable risk factors have been identified. More research into the aetiology of this terrible disease is required to arrest the climb in its incidence.

8

Diseases of the urogenital system

URINARY TRACT INFECTION

Escherichia coli is by far the commonest urinary pathogen, accounting for 80–90% of infections.

The term 'significant bacteriuria' has been introduced to signify the presence of more than 100 000 organisms per ml of urine. Organisms which have multiplied in the bladder before voiding will be present in large numbers (usually more than 100 000 per ml), whereas contaminants are usually less than 100 000 organisms per ml. Although significant bacteriuria is a statistical concept and false negatives may be encountered under conditions of extreme diuresis when bladder emptying is frequent, the demarcation between urinary infection and contamination holds true with few exceptions.

Epidemiology

Along with respiratory infections, infections of the urinary tract are the most common in the population. The prevalence of urinary tract infection in females far exceeds that in males; shortness of the female urethra and bactericidal substances in prostatic secretions are the likely reasons for the difference. Overt infection in women is often precipitated by sexual contact — the so-called 'honeymoon cystitis'.

The prevalence of urinary tract infection in girls of school age is around 1–2% but less than 0.5% in boys. It has been estimated that 5% of girls leaving school have had urinary infection and many of these have radiological abnormalities of the urinary tract. The prevalence of bacteriuria among schoolgirls rises steadily with age, with an annual acquisition rate of 0.32%. A previous history of urinary tract infection can be obtained from a quarter of bacteriuric schoolgirls, compared with about 10% of non-infected controls. Persistence of bacteriuria is more common in girls with vesico-ureteric reflux.

Between the ages of 16 and 65 years, 4% of females and 0.5% of males have significant bacteriuria. Spontaneous remissions and new infections occur at the rate of about 1% of the total female population per annum. The prevalence of significant bacteriuria rises with age and parity, but age is the more powerful factor. Among bacteriuric adult women, 9 out of 10 have a past history of urinary tract infection, compared with two-thirds of matched controls. Nearly 40% of untreated bacteriuric women lose their bacteriuria over a period of a year. These are women in whom the renal tract appears normal on excretion urography. Unlike women, bacteriuria in males is usually associated with a history of recent urinary tract instrumentation.

Bacteriuria is not more common in pregnancy but it rarely remits spontaneously. If untreated, 20% of bacteriuric women will develop acute pyelonephritis but the risk can be largely avoided if the bacteriuria is eradicated by antibacterial therapy. Associations have been reported between bacteriuria in pregnancy and a lowering in mean birthweight, a rise in blood pressure and an increase in perinatal mortality. These have been difficult to substantiate but, if present, they might merely reflect the influence of social class on bacteriuria and birth weight. Since treatment of bacteriuria does not seem to influence these complications, it is likely that it is kidney damage which is the basis of these associations.

There is no evidence that untreated significant bacteriuria in the adult produces progressive kidney damage. In childhood the sequelae may be more serious, e.g. impairment of kidney growth and renal scarring, but further evidence is required on this point.

Prevention

The value of screening for significant bacteriuria in pregnancy is well established since treatment of the bacteriuria largely prevents maternal pyelonephritis. There is no evidence to support screening of schoolchildren or the non-pregnant adult population.

URINARY TRACT CALCULI

Urinary calculi are of two types: bladder stones (which usually occur in boys in developing countries) and renal stones (mostly in men in industrialized societies).

Epidemiology

The prevalence of renal calculi in the UK is about 3%, being more than twice as great in men as in women. The annual incidence has increased throughout the period of observation; for example the hospital discharge rate increased by 50% between 1958 and 1973.

There is a close association between the incidence of renal calculi and the intake of animal protein. This is reflected in the higher incidence in social classes I and II. Renal stone formation appears to be rare in vegetarians.

Prevention

There is laboratory evidence that reducing the animal protein intake reduces the risk of renal stone formation.

ANALGESIC NEPHROPATHY

Chronic ingestion of analgesic mixtures has been shown to be associated with renal papillary necrosis and interstitial nephritis.

Epidemiology

In a number of instances, ingestion of large amounts of phenacetin has been associated with epidemics of renal failure, the best known being in the Swiss watch industry and in a Swedish town called Huskvarna where phenacetin abuse began during the influenza pandemic of 1918–19. Ingestion of phenacetin-containing powders in Huskvarna became habitual and, during the 1940s and 1950s, the mortality from renal failure rose sharply. By 1960, phenacetin use was 10 times greater than in neighbouring towns and deaths from renal failure were five times as common.

Analgesic nephropathy is reported to be particularly prevalent in Australia, being responsible for one-quarter of all renal deaths. In the UK, the disease is less common — about 500 cases of chronic renal failure per year or 1 in 10 of all such cases. The disease is rare under the age of 30, and 80% of cases are in women.

Prevention

In response to the strong circumstantial evidence, phenacetin has been withdrawn from the market in many countries and there is some indication that the incidence of interstitial nephritis has fallen as a result. In individuals suffering from analgesic nephropathy, the avoidance of phenacetin results in striking clinical improvement.

CANCER OF THE KIDNEY

There are two important primary malignancies of the kidney: nephroblastoma (Wilms' tumour) which occurs almost exclusively in children and accounts for 10% of all primary renal neoplasms; and adenocarcinoma which is extremely rare in children.

Epidemiology

Renal cancer accounts for 1% of all malignancies and is a ubiquitous disease showing no marked racial or social class variation. It is responsible for about 2500 cases (1700 deaths) annually in the UK, two-thirds being in men. In both sexes, 90% of cases are over the age of 50 years.

Case–control studies suggest that renal cancer in adults is a disease of cigarette smokers, in whom there is a five-fold increase in risk. Pipe smokers may also be at risk. Other risk factors may include analgesic abuse, renal calculi and Balkan nephropathy (in which there is a 100-fold risk of renal pelvis cancer). These identified risks are at odds with the absence of racial and social class variation.

Prevention

The control of smoking and analgesic abuse would reduce the incidence of this disease. The increased survival of patients with Wilms' tumours in recent years has enabled the identification of genetic factors in this disease. Genetic counselling may be justified in these cases.

CANCER OF THE BLADDER

Bladder cancer is usually a transitional cell carcinoma of the urothelium. Less commonly squamous carcinoma or adenocarcinoma may be found. It is likely that there are two distinct forms — a relatively benign papillary lesion which rarely invades the mucosa and an invasive lesion which is often flat and runs a much more aggressive clinical course. The development of malignant bladder tumours is often preceded by pre-malignant papillomata or carcinoma *in situ*.

Epidemiology

Bladder cancer is the sixth most common cause of cancer mortality in men in the UK following cancer of the lung, stomach, prostate, colon and rectum. It causes about 3000 male deaths per annum and 1300 female deaths. The disease is rare in the young but the death rate rises dramatically after the age of 45 years. Over the past three decades, age-standardized incidence rates appear to have increased only a little in men and to have remained steady in women.

The incidence of bladder cancer is related to social class, with the standardized mortality ratio increasing from 79 in social class I to 115 in class V. The SMR is highest in skilled manual workers (125), probably reflecting occupational factors in disease incidence. A similar, but more marked gradient, is seen in women (who are classified by their husband's occupation). In the UK

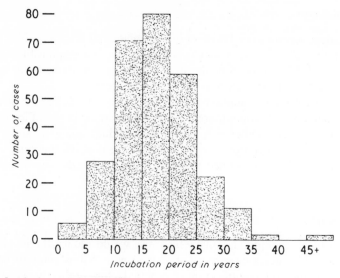

Fig. 8.1 Incubation periods of bladder tumours among dyestuff workers. (Source: Case et al 1954 British Journal of Industrial Medicine 11: 75–104.)

the incidence is highest in parts of West Yorkshire due, it is thought, to the presence of the dye-manufacturing industry. An association with occupational risks has been recognized since 1895 when a high incidence was found among workers producing aniline dyestuffs. The relative risk among dyestuff workers exposed to aromatic amines can be as high as 30 and similar risks have been found in workers in the rubber industry and those involved in the production and insulation of electrical cables. Beta-naphthylamine and benzidine are both potent bladder carcinogens. The monomer of polyvinyl chloride has also been identified as a risk factor. Bladder tumours occur after a long latent period, often more than 20 years (*Fig. 8.1*), and despite the safety measures taken by high-risk industries, further cases of occupational bladder cancer are likely to appear.

The reported incidence is lower in Asian countries than in Europe; in most Eastern European countries it is somewhat lower than in Western Europe. In the US non-white population it is half that in the whites.

The use of tobacco carries a 2–4 fold increased risk of bladder cancer, especially in cigarette smokers, and it appears that there may be a dose–response relationship. An important aetiological factor in developing countries is *Schistosoma haematobium* infection of the bladder.

Prevention

In the UK there are restrictions on the manufacture, import and handling of most known bladder carcinogens. Although not of proven benefit, surveillance of workers at risk using urine cytology is widely practised. The sensitivity of this test in published reports varies from 55% to 100%, with a mean of 72%. Health education about the dangers of cigarette smoking is another important preventive measure.

BENIGN PROSTATIC HYPERTROPHY

The hyperplasia affects glandular, muscular and fibrous tissues in varying degree. It is the effects of obstruction, such as hydronephrosis and renal infection, that are dangerous.

Epidemiology

Some prostatic enlargement begins to develop in most men by the age of 50, and the majority have evidence of hypertrophy by 60 years. By the seventh decade there is disturbance of bladder function in 30% of men, of whom about a third develop severe enough obstruction to require surgical relief. About 10–15% of men are likely to require prostatectomy for benign prostatic hypertrophy.

Half the cases requiring operative treatment are admitted to hospital only when acute retention has supervened; postoperative mortality is 2–3 times as great in emergency cases as in 'cold' cases in whom it is between 2 and 4%.

This very common and debilitating affliction of the ageing man is still poorly understood. The incidence appears to be considerably lower in the yellow races. Previous castration seems to prevent prostatic hypertrophy in men, and an imbalance between androgens and oestrogens may be the causative factor.

Prevention

There are no known preventive measures.

CANCER OF THE PROSTATE

This common disorder of elderly men is usually an adenocarcinoma with a predilection for metastasizing to bone.

Epidemiology

There are almost 5000 deaths a year from prostatic cancer in England and Wales, making this the fourth most common fatal neoplasm in men. In the USA, the disease is even more common and is second only to lung cancer as a cause of death from cancer.

Although extremely uncommon before the age of 50 years, its incidence rises faster with age over 50 years than any other neoplasm. The incidence has doubled in the UK during the last 50 years and the rate is slightly greater in the lower social classes. While prostatic cancer is rare in developing countries, it is twice as common in American black people as in caucasians. The incidence in migrants from low incidence countries rises over two generations.

Evidence from case–control studies suggests that prostatic cancer is, at least partly, a sexually transmitted disease. It is uncommon in unmarried men, three times more common in men with children and particularly common in divorced men. Sufferers are also more likely to give a history of early intercourse, early marriage, use of prostitutes, high sexual appetite and venereal infection. High antibody titres to herpes and cytomegaloviruses indicate a possible viral aetiology. Carefully controlled prospective studies have suggested that patients with benign hypertrophy have a 4–5 fold increased risk of prostatic cancer.

Prevention

Although sexual promiscuity and normal fertility appear to be associated with prostatic cancer, prevention is unlikely to follow this knowledge. More important perhaps is the relationship between benign and malignant prostatic diseases and the possibility that a more aggressive approach to the former might result in a lower incidence of cancer.

CANCER OF THE TESTIS

The seminoma and teratoma are the most important of several histologically distinct tumours of the testis. Their epidemiology, although not identical, is sufficiently similar for them to be considered together.

Epidemiology

Testicular cancer is an uncommon disease with 500 new cases and 200 deaths occurring each year in England, but the incidence is increasing. It has an unusual age distribution in that the incidence declines with age. Thus, although representing only 0.6% of all male cancer deaths, it is the seventh most common cancer in male children and fourth most common in men aged 15–34 years.

Cancer of the testis has some characteristics of a 'new' disease, being rare in non-whites and more common in higher social classes; this class difference has been lessening in recent cohorts. The only important and clearly demonstrated risk factor is an undescended testis which has a 10-fold increase in the risk of malignant change. Attempts to incriminate gonadal mumps have been inconclusive. The age distribution suggests virus infection and androgen dependency as possible factors, while case–control studies incriminate trauma and a family history of gonadal tumours.

Prevention

With the exception of the early detection and correction of undescended testes, there is little at present on which to base effective prevention of testicular cancer.

CANCER OF THE PENIS

There are two forms: a papillary verrucous mass which is a well-differentiated squamous tumour, and an ulcerating poorly differentiated lesion.

Epidemiology

Penile cancer is a rare disease in developed countries, representing less than 0.5% of male cancer and with only 100–150 deaths each year in England. The incidence rises sharply with age. Cancer of the penis is much more common in Africa and Asia; it is the most common of all cancers in Chinese, accounting for 15–20% of cases.

Because of its rarity in developed countries, case–control studies have been necessary to test aetiological hypotheses. A history of phimosis, syphilis or penile warts is more often obtained from cases than controls. The wives of men who develop cancer of the penis have an excess of cervical cancer, suggesting a common infective aetiology. Penile cancer is very rare in circumcised men, especially if circumcision took place before puberty. This may contribute to the low incidence of the disease in social class I.

Prevention

It appears likely that penile hygiene is important in avoiding this rare but distressing disease. Circumcision and the avoidance of genital infection would appear to be effective preventive measures. When circumcision is carried out in the neonatal period, the protection is almost complete; when performed later in childhood, the effect is less marked.

CANCER OF THE OVARY

There are two main types of ovarian cancer: the germ-cell tumour which is most common in young women, and the cystadenocarcinoma which is responsible for most adult cases.

Epidemiology

Cancer of the ovary is the fourth most common fatal neoplasm in women in the UK, there being more than 5000 cases and almost 4000 deaths annually. It is increasing in incidence at the rate of 1% per annum and the incidence has trebled since 1900.

Ovarian cancer is common in developed countries, but rare in the Third World; the incidence is rising fastest in countries where it is still uncommon. Migrant studies suggest that environmental factors are aetiologically important. No significant social class variation has been noted.

The disease is almost twice as common in nulliparous women as in women who have borne children. Impaired fertility has also been noted more often in cases than in controls. Cystadenocarcinoma appears to be related to continuous ovulation, being rare in children and in species of animals that ovulate only occasionally. However, while malignant ovarian disease is most common in the elderly, benign ovarian neoplasms are most common in young adults. Although this description bears some similarity to breast neoplasia, early pregnancy does not confer protection from ovarian cancer. Other risk factors which have been identified in case–control studies include a history of subclinical mumps, peripubertal rubella, severe premenstrual tension, gonadal dysgenesis (only for germ-cell tumours) and hormone replacement therapy after the menopause — although oral contraception may protect, perhaps by causing a cessation of ovulation. A family history of gonadal, breast or gynaecological cancer is found in 40% of cases and the genetic predisposition can be transmitted by both sexes.

Prevention

Although many risk factors have been demonstrated, the cause of ovarian cancer is not known. The strength of the family history association and the fact that most cases occur after the menopause suggests that pre-emptive oophorectomy might be worthwhile in high-risk women.

CANCER OF THE UTERUS

Cancer occurs with almost equal frequency at two sites — the endometrium and the uterine cervix. The latter includes both squamous carcinoma and the relatively uncommon adenocarcinoma.

Epidemiology

Carcinoma of the endometrium occurs principally in post-menopausal women. It is rare under the age of 40 and its peak incidence is around 70 years of age. It is more common in Western countries than in the East. There appears to have been little change in its incidence.

The incidence of endometrial carcinoma is highest in nulliparous women, especially those who are married, and there is an inverse relationship with parity. Very obese women are at increased risk. Primary cancers of the ovary and breast occur with above average frequency in women with endometrial carcinoma. It has been suggested that a high ratio of oestrone to other oestrogen compounds is a cause of endometrial cancer.

Oestrogens used for the relief of menopausal symptoms and the prevention of osteoporosis increase the risk of endometrial cancer. The risk rises with increasing dose and duration of therapy and falls after stopping the treatment.

Typically, endometrial cancer presents with post-menopausal bleeding and it is likely that the clarity of this unexpected sign and the thickness of the surrounding myometrium account for the fact that, in the majority of cases, the disease is still localized to the uterus when it is diagnosed. The prognosis is therefore good and well over half the cases are cured by hysterectomy.

The incidence of invasive cancer of the uterine cervix increases rapidly from the age of 25 to 45, then levels off and falls again after the age of 60. In the UK over the past two decades there has been a decline in both incidence (assessed by registration of new cases) and mortality. This may, in part, be due to screening. However, the mortality rate below the age of 35 has doubled in the past decade and, if this trend continues as the women get older, an increase in mortality rates at older ages can be predicted.

In general, the incidence is highest in Central and South America and there is a decreasing gradient across Europe into Asia, the Far East and South Australasia. However, there are exceptions to this trend; for example, the apparently low incidence in Spain and the high incidence in Denmark and the Federal Republic of Germany.

Cases tend to be of lower social class and, within each class, the husbands tend to be employed in jobs that entail periods away from home. In the USA there are racial differences with a higher proportion of black women among cases than controls and a lower proportion of Jews. Compared with age-matched controls, patients with carcinoma of the cervix are less likely to be single, more likely to be widowed, divorced or separated, to have married early, to have had more pregnancies and to have started child-bearing at a young age. They will have started sexual activity at an earlier age, to have had a greater number of sexual partners and more likely to have had venereal disease. They are less likely than controls to have used occlusive methods of contraception. Male promiscuity is also an important factor.

These associations suggest that in adolescence and during the first pregnancy, the cervical epithelium is particularly metaplastic. The two theories concerning aetiology, both as yet unproven, implicate as carcinogenic agents (1) the herpes simplex virus type 2 and (2) proteins from the sperm head.

Prevention

The avoidance of oestrogen replacement therapy appears to be the only preventive measure for endometrial carcinoma. Health education should stress the importance of seeking early medical advice for post-menopausal bleeding.

Cervical neoplasia seems to follow a progressive course from epithelial dysplasia to carcinoma *in situ* to invasive cancer. The incidence of the earlier stages reached its maximum 15–20 years earlier than that of invasive cancer. It is not possible to predict what proportion of pre-malignant disease will progress to invasion nor to say how many cases of invasive disease go through a recognizable pre-invasive phase. On screening, many more women are found to have epithelial dysplasia and *in situ* carcinoma than would be expected to develop invasive cancer, which suggests that most of these lesions do not progress to the invasive stage or that their incidence has increased.

Unfortunately, there were no randomized control trials of cytological screening for cancer of the cervix when the technique was introduced and it would be unethical to do so now. Studies from Aberdeen, British Columbia, Finland and Iceland have shown that a falling incidence of invasive cancer is related to the intensity of screening. There is a suggestion that in some places mortality from cervical cancer is also falling, but this might be due to improved treatment or other factors such as the number of hysterectomies performed for unconnected diseases.

It has been estimated that the false negative rate of the test is 20%. This implies that a negative test should be followed after a relatively short interval by a second test and possibly a third before settling into a pattern of routine examination at set intervals. Current policy in the UK is to repeat tests at 5 yearly intervals from the age of 20. Studies have shown the initial response to an invitation to be screened is of the order of 50–60% but that it falls off with increasing age and with socioeconomic group, the poorest coming least readily. The response is poorest in the women thought to be most at risk and it is likely that many of the tests that are now done are on those at least risk of the disease.

9

Diseases of the nervous system, sense organs and skin

CEREBRAL PALSY

Cerebral palsy is a disorder of movement and posture resulting from a permanent, non-progressive lesion above the brain stem. The lesion is usually present at birth although the diagnosis is sometimes not made within the first 18 months of life. About a third of cases have hemiplegia and a further third have diplegia. Associated mental handicap is common, about 25% of children having an IQ below 50 and a further 20% an IQ between 50 and 70. However, intellectual impairment is by no means inevitable.

Epidemiology

The prevalence at birth is impossible to assess with any confidence because of the high mortality of affected infants, death often occurring before a firm diagnosis has been made. Further, it appears that transient signs of cerebral palsy are not uncommon. The borderline between severely clumsy and slightly spastic children is difficult to define, particularly for epidemiological purposes. The prevalence of cerebral palsy in British children of school age is between 2 and 3 per 1000. Several studies have attempted to determine whether the prevalence of cerebral palsy has changed over time and the general impression is that, with improvement in medical care, there has been a reduction.

Several large epidemiological studies of cerebral palsy have been reported but, in some, information on antecedent factors has been derived from the mother's history (which may not be reliable) or from incomplete clinical records. In general, there is a small excess of boys among most types of cerebral palsy and an excess of mothers with difficulties in pregnancy and labour, in particular breech presentation. The mothers tend to be at the extremes of the reproductive age span, or having their first baby or a baby of high birth rank, or are themselves in poor health or with poor physique. The secular changes in incidence may be due partly to differences in the types of mothers giving birth.

Low birth weight is an important factor, occurring in about a quarter of all cases; this is about four times the proportion expected in the population. It is in the group of spastics other than hemiplegics, i.e. largely cerebral diplegics, that low birth weight is clearly very important, being present in 40% of the cases. A stormy birth history and fetal distress are unduly common in cerebral palsy, and multiple births are at particular risk. A study reported in 1951 showed that nearly 40% of the athetoids had a history of kernicterus; this is a condition that is now preventable.

In spastic hemiplegia, postnatal factors are also of importance, 17% of cases having followed postnatal disasters such as meningitis. Injury to an infant may also cause spastic hemiplegia or other forms of cerebral palsy.

In Britain, genetic factors do not seem to be of importance except in a small proportion, perhaps 3%. But in countries where inter-marriage between close relatives is common, the proportion of genetically determined cases is much higher.

Prevention

Certain types are almost certainly preventable by excellent obstetric and neonatal care; the prevalence of others will be reduced if the proportion of mothers at high risk by reason of age, parity or ill health falls.

IDIOPATHIC EPILEPSY

It was Hippocrates who first ascribed epilepsy to a disorder of the brain. It is now recognized to be a recurrent disturbance in the chemico-electrical activity of the brain, manifesting itself in a symptom complex in which the essential components are impairment of consciousness, disturbance of the autonomic nervous system, sensory abnormalities and psychic disturbance.

Epidemiology

Determining the prevalence of epilepsy is not easy. There is a diversity of definitions used in epidemiological studies. To be regarded as having epilepsy, the person must have had a fit or have taken regular anticonvulsants, although epidemiological studies differ in the period during which these have occurred.

There is a 100-fold difference in the prevalence rates reported from various studies but these relate to the criteria adopted and the completeness of ascertainment of cases. A review of eight large, well-conducted studies of non-febrile epilepsy in the 10–20 years age group has given a prevalence rate of 4 per 1000. A general practitioner with 2500 patients will have care of 18–20 people with epilepsy, of whom more than half are children. A UK Government report suggested that about 300 000 people in England and Wales have epilepsy, although under 20 000 are registered as disabled.

One in five have their first attack before their first birthday. Grand mal is the commonest presenting type of seizure, affecting half the children. One in six presents with febrile convulsions and the risk of developing epilepsy for children who have experienced febrile convulsions appears to be 3 or 4%.

In three-quarters of cases, there is no known aetiological factor; in the remaining cases, birth hazards, malformations and postnatal factors (infection or accident) have been incriminated.

Two-thirds of epileptic children are educated in normal schools; the remainder, having multiple handicaps (including educational retardation), are in special schools. The progress and future of the child with epilepsy seems to be more dependent on the nature of other physical handicaps than the occurrence of fits.

Genetic factors are generally regarded as important since a family history of epilepsy in first- or second-degree relatives is obtained in about 30% of patients. However, they do not obey simple Mendelian rules.

Prevention

There are no known preventive measures. Genetic counselling for epileptic parents may play a small part in reducing the incidence. Prevention of attacks depends on adequate therapy and the avoidance of precipitating factors.

MULTIPLE SCLEROSIS

In this disease, patches of demyelination occur at different times and in different places throughout the central nervous system. The diagnosis rests on the evidence of multiple lesions. In the early stages there may be complete remission of symptoms. Occasionally it may be steadily progressive from the beginning.

Epidemiology

Studies in the Orkney and Shetland Isles have shown a steady increase in prevalence over the 20 years from 1954 to 1974. The changing age structure of the population is insufficient to account totally for the rise in prevalence; this is attributed to the fact that the patients are not dying (e.g. of infections which at one time led to the death of many patients) at the rate that new cases are emerging. A study in Rochester, Minnesota has shown that while the incidence of the disease has remained constant over 60 years, its prevalence has doubled.

The peak incidence for the disease is around the age of 30. In Britain, it is the commonest cause of disability in the young adult. Almost 60% of cases are in women.

In general, prevalence increases with latitude, rates being low (under 5 per 100 000 population) in the parts of Asia and Africa that have been studied and highest in Orkney and Shetland (309 and 184 per 100 000 respectively). In America, black and Oriental populations have much lower rates than do whites, but they still demonstrate these geographic gradients. However, the relationship with latitude is less clear in Asia and the Pacific countries.

On the whole, migrants retain much of the risk of their place of birth. Prevalence studies of migrants from high- to low-risk areas indicate that those migrating before the age of 15 years acquire the lower risk of their new residence. Migrants from low to high-risk areas in childhood and adolescence increase their risk of multiple sclerosis. These data serve to define multiple sclerosis as an acquired environmental disease whose acquisition in ordinary circumstances takes place years before the clinical onset. They point to an infective (probably viral) cause for multiple sclerosis. There is also evidence that genetic factors are involved. Family studies show that about 10% of patients have an affected relative; twin studies also point to the influence of genetic factors. The genetic influence seems to be related to the HLA system.

Prevention

There are no known preventive measures.

MIGRAINE

The three features that are usually considered most characteristic of migraine are: (1) the unilateral distribution of the headache; (2) the accompanying nausea or actual vomiting; and (3) some warning that the attack is coming, typically a visual disturbance.

Epidemiology

Only about half of those with migraine consult their doctor because of their headaches; the proportion who consult a neurologist is even lower. Patients with migraine who consult a doctor may be different in a number of respects from those who do not consult a doctor; it has been shown that the intelligent migraine sufferer is more likely to consult a doctor. This points to the desirability of screening whole populations and not relying on general practice consultations in studying incidence and prevalence.

The diagnosis of migraine depends largely on symptoms and, in attempting to measure its prevalence, it is appropriate to screen the population using a questionnaire. The prevalence of migraine in the previous year is highest in young adults of both sexes; in all age groups it is higher in women than in men. Approximate prevalence rates are: age 21–34 — men 20%, women 30%; age 35–54 — men 17%, women 26%.

Epidemiological studies do not provide support for the widely held views that sufferers from migraine are more likely to be intelligent or of high social class. Where the prevalence has been reported as highest in classes I and II, this is probably due to the fact that subjects were asked whether or not they had had migraine, and this self-diagnosis is likely to have introduced a serious bias.

A number of studies have suggested that there is no primary relationship between migraine, epilepsy and allergy, but in one study migraine sufferers reported bilious attacks, travel sickness and eczema more often than other groups.

Prevention

There are no known preventive measures for the community as a whole but individuals can prevent attacks by avoiding any precipitating factors known to them.

PARKINSON'S DISEASE

The Shaking Palsy (paralysis agitans) was first described by James Parkinson in 1817. It is characterized by a combination of rigidity, tremor and brady-kinesia. The pathological cause is a degeneration of the globus pallidus and substantia nigra.

Epidemiology

The disease usually develops in late middle age. Secular trends for age-specific mortality rates for paralysis agitans in England and Wales show that among men aged 75–84 there has been an increase in mortality, but among younger men a decrease; the younger the age group the greater the relative decline. The picture is somewhat similar for women. Despite the difficulties associated with analyses based solely on death certification data, it seems like-ly that there has been a real increase over time in the age of onset of Parkin-son's disease.

The epidemics of encephalitis lethargica that occurred mainly between 1918 and 1926 were followed by the emergence of post-encephalitic Parkin-sonism. The analysis of paralysis agitans mortality by cohorts lends support to the view that a majority of cases of Parkinson's disease up to the present may be post-encephalitic in origin. If it is true that clinically defined idiopathic Parkinson's disease may be a very late result of a viral infection, then new cases may be the end result of infection that has been unrecognized clinically. New epidemics of viral infection could be responsible for an upsurge in the occurrence of Parkinson's disease.

Prevention

There are no known preventive measures.

PRIMARY MALIGNANT TUMOURS OF THE BRAIN

The usual histological types are the medulloblastoma and astrocytoma, which are the common types in children, and the glioblastoma which accounts for 50% of adult cases.

Epidemiology

Brain tumours are generally underdiagnosed; they are present in about 1% of autopsies and may represent up to 9% of all primary neoplasms. The overall incidence of brain cancer in most countries is aroung 50 per million. Thus there are about 3000 cases in the UK each year, with 2500 deaths. The incidence is about 20 per million throughout childhood. Cancer registration data suggest that the incidence of brain tumours is falling by about 1% per annum. There is no marked geographical variation in the incidence.

There is an excess of male cases (1.5:1) and the peak incidence is at ages 55–74 years. The male excess in children (1.7:1) is entirely due to medulloblastoma. There is no clear social class variation in mortality.

Epidemiological studies have given few clues to the aetiology of cerebral tumours. One exception is the high incidence noted in farm residents, suggesting an infective cause. Serological evidence supports an association with toxoplasma infection and animal experiments have implicated some viruses.

Prevention

Further knowledge of aetiology is required before effective primary prevention can be offered. Secondary prevention is based on early detection, the most usual indicator being epilepsy. The prevalence of brain tumours in epileptic patients varies between 2 and 15%. A change in the nature of the attacks, loss of control of the disease and a late age of onset are suggestive signs.

SENILE CATARACT

Cataract is defined as any opacity in the lens. It is due to degeneration of lens fibres, either the result of coagulation of proteins primarily in the cortex or due to slow sclerosis in the nucleus. Cataract becomes visually significant when the location and degree are sufficient to degrade the retinal image. Congenital cataract (as occurs in the rubella syndrome) is not considered here.

Epidemiology

About three in every 1000 of the British population are registered as blind or partially sighted — but registration is believed to underestimate the true prevalence of blindness by about 30% and rather more for partial sight. Senile cataract accounts for 5% of certified cases of blindness.

It is rare in persons under 50, unless associated with some metabolic disturbance such as diabetes, but it is almost universal to some degree in persons over 70. It occurs equally in men and women, is usually bilateral but often develops earlier in one eye than the other.

There is considerable genetic influence in its incidence and in hereditary cases it may appear at an earlier age in successive generations. Compared with age-matched controls, cataract patients have a higher prevalence of glaucoma and a higher level of blood pressure.

Prevention

There are no known preventive measures. Regular examination of the eyes is worthwhile for all people over 65 and, although some have macular degeneration for which there is no treatment, many can be helped, for example by improved lighting, glasses and low vision aids. Operative treatment of senile cataract often leads to a dramatic improvement in the sight.

CHRONIC GLAUCOMA

The glaucomas are a group of diseases sharing in common a characteristic appearance of the optic nerve head (glaucomatous cupping) and visual field defects. Four-fifths have a raised intraocular pressure. Primary adult glaucomas are of two types: open angle glaucoma associated with obstruction in the trabecular meshwork, and closed angle glaucoma in which contact between the iris and the trabecular meshwork blocks its openings. The chronic forms of glaucoma tend to be insidious in onset, slowly progressive and commonest in the elderly; they lead to blindness if untreated.

Epidemiology

Chronic glaucoma is one of the principal cause of visual loss throughout the world; in Britain it accounts for over 12% of registered blindness.

The mean intraocular pressure in the population is about 15 mm Hg but its distribution is not symmetrical, being slightly skewed towards high pressures. In glaucoma the pressure is usually over 20 mm Hg and may rise to 30 mm Hg or more. About 10% of people over the age of 40 have pressures greater than 20 mm Hg. In the UK about 1% of people aged 40 years and over, and about 5% of those over 65, develop glaucoma. The proportion is even higher (about 10%) by the age of 80. There is little difference between the sexes.

Over the age of 40, 3% of the population have significantly raised intraocular pressures but without evidence of glaucoma, i.e. there are no optic nerve or visual field changes. Over 10 years about 10% of 'ocular hypertensives' develop glaucoma with field loss but it is not possible to identify the potential glaucoma patient before the development of a field defect. The risk of developing glaucoma rises with the intraocular pressure.

Glaucoma is, in part at least, genetically determined and the prevalence is around 10% in the first-degree relatives of known cases. In the USA the prevalence is three times as great in black people as in caucasians.

Prevention

Untreated glaucoma is a severe threat to sight but, if discovered early and well managed, the prospects for the preservation of vision are very good. Reducing the pressure is most effective in those cases with only slight visual field loss, so that early diagnosis is important. Between two-thirds and three-quarters of cases of glaucoma remain undiagnosed.

Tonometry as a screening procedure fails to identify a significant proportion of those with glaucoma and produces a large number of subjects who are asymptomatic, have normal visual fields and are distinguished from the rest of the population only by the fact that their pressure is statistically abnormal. Follow-up studies have shown that the majority of these do not develop detectable loss of vision from glaucoma. It would be undesirable to treat them as a preventive measure, especially as the treatment itself may have undesirable side effects. The incidence of false positive results is much less in screening visual fields than in tonometry.

General practitioners are well placed to identify asymptomatic patients with glaucoma. They see a high proportion of the elderly patients under their care, especially those with the risk factors of hypertension and diabetes, and ophthalmoscopy would identify most early glaucomas.

The first-degree relatives of glaucoma patients should be screened by an ophthalmologist or ophthalmic optician every few years after the age of 35.

XEROPHTHALMIA

This is due to vitamin A deficiency, and the eye is the only organ characteristically affected in man. Impairment of rod function leads to night blindness and later the conjunctiva undergoes the changes of sclerosis (drying, thickening, wrinkling, pigmentation and loss of wetability).

Epidemiology

Xerophthalmia remains the major cause of blindness in many developing countries. It mainly affects children under the age of 4 years when dietary intake of vitamin A has been grossly inadequate for a long time. Nearly all children with xerophthalmia have evidence of protein energy malnutrition.

Prevention

In areas where xerophthalmia is a problem, vitamin A fortification of such foodstuffs as cereal grains, sugar or tea should be considered. Young children may be protected by six-monthly doses of vitamin A: 100 000 international units under 1 year and 200 000 i.u. at 1–6 years.

DEAFNESS

There is a very small number of children who are born deaf because the conducting apparatus has failed to develop in part or in whole. The causes of congenital deafness include perinatal problems (anoxia, haemolytic disease of the newborn), rubella in pregnancy and hereditary deafness.

Acquired sensori-neural deafness is due to 'trauma' which may be a head injury, pressure changes affecting the inner ear such as blasts or explosions, and exposure to excessive noise such as 'pop music'. Presbyacusis (senile deafness) is another form of acquired sensori-neural deafness; the term usually applies to that type of progressive deafness which comes on and advances for no apparent reason with the years. It is most commonly noticed around the age of 60 but a premature onset may be associated with bouts of otitis media in childhood or with prolonged exposure to noise throughout the working life.

Conductive deafness may be due to injuries or inflammation of the middle ear, otosclerosis and affections of the external auditory canal (wax, foreign bodies, otitis externa, atresia or tumours).

Epidemiology

One child per thousand is born profoundly deaf, and the prevalence of moderate and lesser degrees of hearing deficit is several times as great. Among school entrants, inspection has revealed definite hearing defects in 8 per thousand while further observation was required for 18 per thousand. The prevalence of deafness increases with age. In a survey of elderly people (over

75 years of age) 9% were effectively totally deaf. Many more could hear only the shouted voice and were prepared to tolerate the disability without seeking help.

Prevention

Deafness associated with maternal rubella or haemolytic disease of the newborn is now preventable, the first by rubella immunization of girls and the latter by the administration of anti-D serum. Occupational deafness is prevented by reducing the noise level of industrial processes and, when appropriate, providing ear protectors for workers.

Screening tests of hearing are carried out routinely at 6–9 months. Babies with serious hearing defects need early auditory stimulation if they are to speak normally; poor hearing can lead to educational retardation.

ACNE VULGARIS

Acne is caused by a defect in the sebaceous glands which leads to the production of large quantities of sebum. This seborrhoea is primarily androgen induced and may represent a (possibly genetic) hyper-responsiveness of the sebaceous glands to circulating androgens. Other aetiological factors are involved, in particular blockage of the pilosebaceous duct and subsequent colonization with *Propionibacterium acnes*, *Staphylococcus epidermis* and *Pityrosporum ovale*.

Epidemiology

Acne is an almost universal problem of adolescence. At 14–19 years, three-quarters of boys and two-thirds of girls have comedones and at least two papules on the face and neck; 15% of adolescents with acne have a condition of sufficient severity to warrant advice from a doctor. Because of the earlier onset of puberty in girls, acne is generally seen earlier in them than in boys, reaching its peak incidence and severity by the time they are aged between 16 and 17 years; whereas the maximum incidence and severity in boys are between 17 and 19 years. The incidence and severity then decline gradually.

In the age group 17–24 years, the prevalence of acne is greatest in social classes I and II; over 25 it is more common in class V. The condition worsens in the premenstrual phase and a higher prevalence of dysmenorrhoea has been reported in acne patients. There is no outstanding evidence to incriminate food as a causal factor. A strong genetic influence exists in acne, with a high degree of concordance in identical twins.

Prevention

There are no known methods for the prevention of acne. Treatment aims to prevent the disease from progressing and to prevent psychological trauma and dermal scarring.

CANCER OF THE SKIN

Occupational skin cancer

Cancer of the scrotum was the first instance of occupational malignancy to be recognized. In 1775, Percival Pott (a surgeon at St. Bartholomew's Hospital, London) described the occurrence of scrotal cancer in chimney sweeps. Since Pott's day, skin cancer has been observed to occur at other sites, most usually on exposed skin surfaces. It has been recorded in men working with pitch and tar, with arsenic, and in those exposed to mineral oils. In the early decades of this century, cancer of the scrotum was occurring in cotton-mule spinners as a result of the shale oil lubricant penetrating the workers' clothing as they leaned over a horizontal bar 3 feet above the floor. More recently men exposed to cutting oils in the engineering industry have been found to be at risk of skin cancer. The carcinogens in pitch, tar and oil are considered to be polycyclic aromatic hydrocarbons. In the early days of radiography, many radiologists unwittingly exposed themselves to high doses of X-rays which produced malignant changes in their skin.

Basal cell carcinoma

This is the most common form of skin cancer. Lesions are usually on the face of the middle aged or elderly. Cumulative exposure to sunlight is the most important factor and the tumour is most prevalent in white people living near the equator. Photosensitizing pitch, tar and oils can act as co-carcinogens with ultraviolet radiation. Previous treatment with arsenic, once present in many 'tonics', may predispose to multiple basal carcinomata, often after a lag of many years. Interestingly, the distribution of tumours does not correlate exactly with those areas receiving most sun, e.g. lesions occur commonly on the eyelids, at the inner canthus and behind the ears, but seldom on the back of the hands. The cure rate is over 95%; local recurrence sometimes occurs.

Malignant melanoma

Malignant changes sometimes occur in a pre-existing naevus or in the basal layers of the epidermis. It is an uncommon condition in the UK but the incidence is high in places where fair-skinned people are exposed to too much sunlight, such as Australia and New Zealand. Within the UK the highest rates occur in the South; they are increasing in most regions.

Women have a higher incidence of the condition than men. There is some evidence that oral contraceptives may increase the risk of malignant melanoma in high-risk areas. Mortality is higher in social class I than in class V; this is the reverse of the gradient seen in most other diseases. Survival rates are higher in women than in men.

Prevention

Workers at risk through occupational exposure to pitch, tar and mineral oil should be made aware of the danger of the substances with which they are working and encouraged to report any suspicious lesions. Protective clothing and good washing facilities are essential. Machines on which cutting oils are used are now guarded to prevent splashing. Only oils of low carcinogenicity should be used. Exposure to diagnostic X-rays is controlled by the use of shields, and protective clothing. Fair-skinned people living in the tropics can reduce their exposure to ultraviolet light by suitable clothing and the use of some barrier creams.

10

Diseases of bones and joints

Anatomical and physiological derangements of the skeletal system constitute a common health problem worldwide. Although not a major cause of death, they are responsible for much suffering, physical handicap, absence from work and demand on health services.

OSTEOPOROSIS

There is a continuing debate as to whether osteoporosis is a disease entity or merely a consequence of ageing. However, it is convenient to regard osteoporosis as the pathological consequence, in terms of pain or fracture, of osteopaenia ('thin bones'). These effects are closely related to absolute bone mass, and it is acceptable to regard all those with significantly less bone than young adults as osteoporotic.

Epidemiology

Men start adult life with more bone than do women. Men lose bone more slowly and so, at all ages, osteoporosis is more common in women than in men. The prevalence of osteoporosis increases steadily with age; it is certainly very common in elderly men, but is universal in elderly women.

Osteoporosis is rare before the menopause. Bone is lost at a faster rate during the 3 years following the menopause than at any other time, regardless of the age at menopause and whether it is natural or artificial. After this initial period of brisk bone loss, further decline in bone volume continues at a reduced rate. The striking association between rapid bone loss and the menopause suggests that oestrogen deficiency is an important factor in osteoporosis. An increasing calcium requirement after the menopause suggests that, in old age, dietary lack of calcium contributes to bone loss.

Racial factors in osteoporosis represent an intriguing paradox for, although bone mass is lower in black people, osteoporotic fractures are rare.

Prevention

Postmenopausal oestrogen deficiency can be avoided by replacement therapy, although the potential hazards (neoplastic and thrombotic) of exogenous oestrogen must be borne in mind. Dietary supplements of calcium or vitamin D can reduce osteoporosis.

POSTMENOPAUSAL FRACTURES

There are three bony injuries which are usually regarded as being associated with osteoporosis, namely the vertebral crush fracture, fracture of the distal forearm (Colles' fracture) and fracture of the proximal femur. These fractures have in common a low incidence before the menopause and a high incidence after the menopause.

Vertebral crush fracture

This is a radiological diagnosis in which the central feature is the absence of trauma.

Epidemiology

After excluding malignant disease (myeloma and metastases), the prevalence of vertebral crush fractures in women is 2.5% at age 60 and 7.5% at age 80. Wedging of vertebrae is a much more common radiological finding than crush fracture, being present in 50% of women aged 75. Little is known of the prevalence of crush fractures in men except that it is lower than in women. Crush fractures are probably less common in black people.

Fracture of the distal forearm

Simultaneous fracture of the distal radius and ulna (Colles' fracture) usually results from a fall in which the person lands on an outstretched arm.

Epidemiology

Our knowledge of the epidemiology of wrist fractures relies largely on the results of two studies (one in Oxford and Dundee, the other in Malmo) involving the detailed analysis of accident department records. They both show a striking increase in the incidence of wrist fracture in women between the ages of 40 and 60 years (*Fig. 10.1*).

Wrist and vertebral crush fractures are associated with loss of trabecular bone; it is not surprising, therefore, that there is considerable overlap between the crush fracture population and the wrist fracture population. Of the

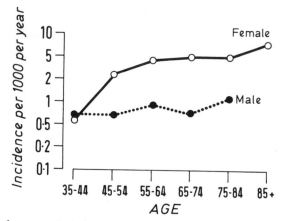

Fig. 10.1 Wrist fractures—the incidence by age and sex.

15% of women who fracture a wrist by the age of 80, one in four has also had a vertebral crush fracture.

Fracture of the proximal femur

This injury is usually termed 'fractured neck of femur' but the diagnosis includes subcapital, transcervical, basal and intertrochanteric fractures.

Epidemiology

Unlike the fractures mentioned above, fracture of the proximal femur almost always results in hospital admission and it has a significant fatality. Routine data can, therefore, be used for epidemiological studies, provided that the inaccuracies inherent in hospital discharge data are borne in mind. Because of its high incidence, high fatality and social consequences, this fracture has been studied more than any other.

In the Western world, femoral neck fracture constitutes the most common cause of death from falls, there being over 2000 such deaths annually in the UK; 80% are in women, mostly over the age of 75. More than 5000 hospital beds are being occupied at any time by patients with a femoral neck fracture.

The classic epidemiological features of femoral neck fracture are shown in *Figure 10.2*. These are:

1. The changing sex incidence, with females predominating after the menopause.
2. The logarithmic increase in incidence with age.
3. Over the age of 85, an incidence of 1% per annum in men and 2% in women.

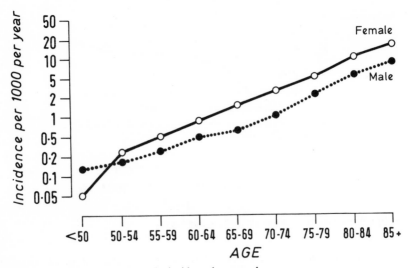

Fig. 10.2 Femoral neck fractures—the incidence by age and sex.

The incidence of femoral neck fracture increases with the distance from the equator; it is uncommon in non-white populations, even in migrants.

It is unlikely that osteoporosis alone explains the increase in incidence with age. Osteomalacia has been found in 40% of these patients in Leeds; barbiturate consumption and cerebrovascular disease have also been implicated.

Prevention

Evidence is accumulating that oestrogen replacement therapy can prevent not only osteoporosis, but also the three kinds of fracture described above. However, it has not yet been shown whether vitamin D supplementation reduces the risk of fracture.

OSTEOMALACIA

Osteomalacia is the clinical syndrome resulting from vitamin D deficiency in adults. They key diagnostic feature is a disturbance in bone mineralisation. The disease can be due to (1) a lack of vitamin D, both exogenous (dietary) and endogenous (produced by the effect of ultraviolet radiation on 7-dehydrocholesterol in the skin); (2) disease of the gastrointestinal tract, kidney or liver; and (3) drugs, such as barbiturates.

Epidemiology

The development of a reproducible assay of plasma vitamin D metabolites has enabled large epidemiological surveys of vitamin D status to be performed. Plasma vitamin D levels give an indication of risk, but only a bone biopsy provides irrefutable diagnostic evidence.

In the UK, osteomalacia is most common in Asian immigrants and in housebound elderly people. Both groups have a low dietary vitamin D intake and a relative or absolute lack of exposure to ultraviolet rays. Blood surveys in Leeds and Bradford have shown biochemical evidence of vitamin D deficiency in 50% of pregnant Asian women, 40% of Asian schoolchildren (in spring) and 40% of housebound caucasian women. Among Asians, vitamin D deficiency appears to be more common in the culturally traditional groups.

Prevention

In the absence of underlying disease (e.g. of the kidney or liver), osteomalacia can be prevented by an adequate intake of vitamin D. However, the vitamin D content of the British and Asian diets is generally low, so that most of the body's vitamin D is produced by the effect of sunlight on the skin. Hence the highest prevalence of vitamin D deficiency at the end of the winter. We believe that in the UK vitamin D supplements should be offered to all housebound people, pregnant Asian women and Asian children.

RICKETS

Rickets is the name given to the clinical syndrome resulting from severe vitamin D deficiency in children.

Epidemiology

Cases of severe rickets were common in poorly nourished children in Scottish and northern cities until the early years of this century (*Fig. 10.3*). Rickets was always less common in the south and in rural areas. The widespread distribution of vitamin D fortified welfare foods and vitamin D supplements led to the almost total disappearance of rickets in the UK by the 1960s. However, sporadic cases continued to occur in poorly nourished children and, more recently, rickets and subclinical vitamin D deficiency have been seen most often in Asian children.

Several blood surveys have been performed which describe the spectrum of biochemical vitamin D deficiency. By late winter, it affects over one-third of the Asian children examined in Bradford but rickets itself remains uncommon. Reported cases occur more commonly in girls. Low dietary vitamin D

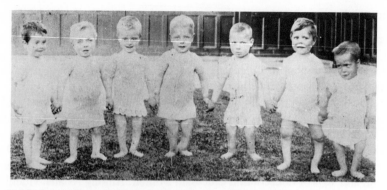

Fig. 10.3 Rickets in Glasgow children in the early years of the century.

and limited exposure to ultraviolet rays in sunlight both contribute to the aetiology of rickets in Asians; much subclinical vitamin D deficiency is spontaneously cured by sunlight during the summer months.

Prevention

As with osteomalacia, rickets can be prevented by vitamin D supplements. It is worth noting that rickets is rare in breastfed children. Powdered milk (but not cows' milk) is fortified with vitamin D and supplements may be necessary after weaning.

PAGET'S DISEASE OF BONE (OSTEITIS DEFORMANS)

This is a disease of unknown aetiology whose main clinical features are bone pain, deafness and high output cardiac failure. As it is often asymptomatic, diagnosis is based on radiographic appearances and a raised serum alkaline phosphatase.

Epidemiology

Large radiological surveys in Britain indicate a prevalence of more than 5% in people over 50. The annual crude death rate associated with the disease in England is about 3 per million. Age- and sex-specific death rates show higher rates in men than in women but death rates have decreased steadily in cohorts born since 1880, the fall being greater in men. Mortality from malignant tumours of bone, which in the elderly are often a consequence of Paget's disease, follows a similar pattern.

Hospital discharges for Paget's disease are more common in those parts of the UK where rickets was prevalent at the end of the last century, suggesting that vitamin D deficiency in childhood may contribute to the pathogenesis of Paget's disease in later life.

Paget's disease appears to be more common in the UK than in the other countries where it has been studied. Although rare in Africans, it is common in American black people, suggesting that both heredity and environment have aetiological roles.

Prevention

Paget's disease may be declining in incidence before the problem of aetiology has been solved. At present, no specific preventive measures can be recommended.

CANCER OF BONE

There are several histologically distinct malignant neoplasms of bone, the most common being osteogenic sarcoma and chondrosarcoma.

Epidemiology

Primary bone cancer is uncommon; there are about 600 new cases each year in the UK with 500 deaths. The overall incidence of primary bone cancer is 8 per million. While it is most common in the elderly (60 per million over 75), there is also a small incidence peak after puberty. This peak, which occurs at 15 years in girls and 18 in boys, is due to osteogenic sarcoma. The incidence of chondrosarcoma increases steadily with age and is especially common in those with multiple exostoses (an autosomal dominant trait). At all ages, primary bone cancer is more common in males, especially in children where the male:female ratio approaches 2:1 for Ewing's sarcoma and osteogenic sarcoma of the long bones.

The major known risk factors for osteogenic sarcoma are bone-seeking radioisotopes and Paget's disease of bone. An interesting and historically important example of the dangers of radioactive substances occurred during and shortly after the First World War when women employed in the luminizing industry developed sarcoma of bone, necrosis of the jaw and aplastic anaemia. In the course of applying luminous paint (containing sulphates of radium mesothorium and radiothorium) to the figures of clocks and watches and certain parts of the machinery of aeroplanes, the workers introduced the paint into their mouths through the habit of pointing the brush between their lips.

It has been estimated that Paget's disease increases the risk of osteogenic sarcoma 30-fold over the age of 40 and that 'Paget's sarcoma' is responsible for 18% of all primary bone cancer, and 50% over the age of 60.

Prevention

The control of occupational exposure to irradiation has been an important sequel to the epidemiologically demonstrated association between ^{223}Ra and osteogenic sarcoma. Paget's disease of bone, the cause of which is unknown, is the single most important factor in bone cancer but it is not yet clear whether treatment of Paget's disease with calcitonin will influence the risk of neoplasm.

ARTHRITIS

Although the arthritides are common health problems, their relatively non-fatal nature and limited use of inpatient resources make routine data poor indicators of prevalence. Most data come from the rather imprecise proxies of self-reporting and sickness absence statistics, or from cumbersome and expensive population surveys. One per cent of the adult population is appreciably handicapped as a result of arthritis and rheumatism. These conditions are responsible for 15% of all immobility and 28% of all disability in the UK. According to the General Household Survey, 30% of the population report aching limbs during a 1-month period, but only 15% of the population consult a doctor with a rheumatic complaint each year. The spectrum of such cases seen in a year in an average general practice of 2500 patients would be as follows:

Muscular aches	110
Lumbar pain	66
Osteoarthosis	63
Trauma	52
Disc lesion	15
Rheumatoid arthritis	13
Gout	4
Sciatica	4
Other	40

Over 70% of hospital rheumatology outpatients have specific clinical syndromes such as rheumatoid arthritis or gout, but the majority of spells of sickness are due to non-specific causes.

RHEUMATOID ARTHRITIS

This is a chronic, non-suppurative, symmetrical, mainly peripheral, inflammatory polyarthritis of synovial joints with associated non-articular features. It is probably a disease of modern times having been first described in 1800.

Epidemiology

Although hospitalization for rheumatoid arthritis is common compared with the other arthritides, the majority of sufferers remain in the community. Despite considerable observer variation, a classification of rheumatoid arthritis devised by the American Rheumatology Association has enabled large-scale epidemiological studies to be performed worldwide with a high degree of comparability.

Rheumatoid arthritis is one of the major causes of physical handicap in the UK. It is estimated that 135 000 adults are affected; it has a prevalence of 3% in women and 1% in men. The difference between the sexes is less marked in the elderly. The modal age of onset is 30 years. There are 25 000 hospital admissions due to rheumatoid arthritis each year in England alone and 1000 deaths.

In other countries the prevalence varies widely, from 0.4% in Japan to 11% in Jamaica, as does the sex ratio (female/male), from 0.5 in West Germany to 13.8 in Japan. However, national mortality data show much less variation, suggesting that the disease is evenly distributed throughout the world.

HLA DW4 is found more often than expected in patients with rheumatoid arthritis, and HLA DW3 may be associated with erosive disease. Rheumatoid arthritis is 15 times more common in people who have a positive rheumatoid factor (RF), but only 25% of RF positive people have rheumatoid arthritis.

Prevention

The failure to identify specific environmental risk factors has so far mediated against effective preventive measures.

OSTEOARTHROSIS

The disease is sometimes local, involving a single joint such as the knee, and sometimes general with many joints involved and the diagnostic sign of Heberden's nodes. It is likely that the final radiological and clinical appearances of the osteoarthritic joint represent the result of more than one pathological process.

Epidemiology

The lack of agreement on what constitutes osteoarthrosis has proved a major obstruction to epidemiological studies. While mortality and hospital data can be a guide to the importance of osteoarthrosis in relation to other conditions, the wide variations in classification and diagnostic criteria have proved a disincentive to epidemiologists. However, clinical studies have been of value in highlighting some risk factors.

Although there are 35 000 hospital admissions annually for this disease, most patients remain entirely in the community. In Britain, osteoarthrosis is the most common cause of physical handicap, more than half of those so handicapped being elderly women. Of the 400 deaths attributed annually to osteoarthrosis in the UK, 300 are in women. This closely reflects the sex distribution of the disease.

While the disease in men is often localized, affecting large proximal joints, it is usually generalized and peripheral in women. The prevalence of osteoarthrosis of the hip in women aged over 65 is of the order of 5–10%. The relative absence of the disease in the ankles is interesting, and it may be due to biomechanical factors resulting in lower stresses on the joints and more stability.

Although osteoarthrosis is more common in the elderly, it is not exclusively a result of ageing. Risk factors identified clinically include congenital dislocation of the hip; trauma (intra-articular fracture, neuropathic joints, torn menisci); metabolic diseases (acromegaly, haemoglobinopathies); post-inflammation (rheumatoid arthritis, sepsis, gout); and haemorrhage (haemophilia).

The specific disease marker of Heberden's nodes may be more common in Europeans and familial aggregation of these nodes points to a genetic factor.

Interestingly, osteoarthrosis of the hip and fracture of the femoral neck hardly ever coincide.

Prevention

The minority of cases in whom specific risk factors are identified offer some scope for prevention. In particular, screening for congenital dislocation of the hip and early treatment should remove that cause. For the great majority, there are no known preventive measures.

ANKLYOSING SPONDYLITIS

This is an inflammatory arthritis of the spine which, characteristically, involves the sacro-iliac joints.

Epidemiology

Most of our knowledge of the epidemiology of ankylosing spondylitis has been gathered from clinical observations. It is predominantly a disease of young adults and until recently it was thought to be confined to men, with a prevalence of 1 in 2500. However, a survey of 'healthy' blood donors possessing HLA B27 revealed radiological and/or clinical evidence of ankylosing spondylitis in both men and women. The true prevalence is probably higher than had been thought.

It is rare in non-caucasians but, even in those populations who have a low prevalence of both HLA B27 and ankylosing spondylitis, the close association between the two still exists. This genetic link is central to the aetiology of ankylosing spondylitis; 95% of cases possess HLA B27 and 35% of their first-degree relatives who possess HLA B27 develop the disease, compared with only 2% of those without HLA B27.

However, environmental factors also play a part. Discordance in twin studies suggests an environmental role in the initial development and in the severity of the disease.

Prevention

Although nothing can be done to influence the possession of HLA B27, the interrelation between genetic and environmental factors raises hope for the possible prevention of this inherited disease.

GOUT

Gout is an acute inflammatory arthritis, usually associated with an inborn error of metabolism resulting in an excess of uric acid in the blood (hyperuricaemia) and soft tissues.

Epidemiology

Gout occurs in almost all human communities. In caucasians, the prevalence is just under 1% but, in pigmented peoples, the prevalence varies from zero in South African Bantu to 2% in New Zealand Maoris. The annual incidence of gout in Britain is about 1 per 1000 and it is most common in social class I.

The disease is 5–10 times more common in men than in women; it is rare in prepubertal males and very uncommon in premenopauusal women. However, of the 30 deaths from gout each year in England one-third are in women, suggesting that gout is underdiagnosed in women during life.

The serum uric acid is a normally distributed variable, rising with age, muscle bulk and body weight. It is higher in males, in urban dwellers and in the upper social classes. Hyperuricaemia is found in up to 7% of British men but clinical gout occurs in only 1 in 10 of these. In the elderly, much hyperuricaemia, and at least 10% of cases of gout, are secondary to either drug therapy (such as thiazide diuretics) or to disease (such as leukaemia).

Prevention

Although the basic biochemical derangement is inborn, the clinical syndrome of gout is dependent on environmental factors of which diet is probably the most important. Avoidance of purine-rich foods can contribute to secondary prevention.

11

Endocrine disorders

DIABETES MELLITUS

Diabetes mellitus is characterized by a chronically elevated blood glucose concentration and the disease may vary in its expression from totally asymptomatic to rapidly lethal. Many pathogenic processes have the effect of provoking hyperglycaemia but, in all cases, impaired production or hindrance of the action of insulin is the ultimate mechanism in diabetes mellitus. Diabetes is now classified into insulin dependent (IDDM) and non-insulin-dependent diabetes mellitus (NIDDM).

Epidemiology

The disease is very rare among primitive societies but widespread (a prevalence as high as 7%) in developed countries. War and dietary restrictions stop the appearance of new cases, while periods of prosperity and abundant food increase the number of cases. The disease has appeared rapidly among Jewish immigrants to Israel with its Western culture. Evidence for the protective effect of exercise comes from the deterioriation in glucose tolerance with bedrest, its reversibility afterwards, and the appearance of new cases of diabetes during enforced restriction of exercise (e.g. elderly people kept indoors by bad weather and amputees in wheelchairs).

The age at which the disease is first recognized ranges from early childhood to old age; half the cases are first diagnosed over the age of 50 years. The incidence is similar in both sexes but the case-fatality rate is higher in women.

An oral glucose-tolerance test is said to be normal if the fasting value does not exceed 110 mg per 100 ml in capillary blood, the 2-hour level 120 mg per 100 ml, and for other points in the test 160 mg per 100 ml. A simple capillary or venous blood glucose above 160 mg per 100 ml is regarded as diagnostic if it accords with other clinical features. In a survey of a sample of the Bedford population in 1962, 9–12% of adults had levels above 120 mg per 100 ml and 7% above 140 mg per 100 ml. It is estimated that the prevalence of diabetes in the UK is 3–4% of the adult population, of whom only a third are recognized cases. Many of the previously undiagnosed diabetics in the Bedford study had symptoms of diabetes, or its complications, which were not recognized as such by the sufferers.

'Impaired glucose tolerance' is a term which recognizes the existence of a zone of diagnostic uncertainty. The justification for distinguishing it is based on long-term follow-up studies which show that annually 2–4% of patients in this group develop unequivocal diabetes. There is also the likelihood that some will revert, apparently spontaneously, to normal tolerance. The risk of developing clinically significant diabetic retinopathy in this IGT group has been shown to be virtually nil but, in contrast, they share with unequivocal diabetics a doubling of the risk of coronary heart disease.

There is an increased frequency of certain HLA types in IDDM and of complete HLA identity between diabetic siblings in families where more than one member is affected. Viral infection appears to be the most probable agent linking genetic susceptibility with beta-cell damage and failure. Underlying genetic susceptibility seems to play an even more important role in NIDDM. Almost all affected identical twin pairs are concordant for the disease, compared with about 50% for IDDM. Obesity is a major factor capable of unmasking an underlying NIDDM susceptibility. In some highly inbred and very obese groups (e.g. Pima American Indians, Nauruan Micronesians) over 50% of the population become diabetic by 60 years of age. No single component of nutrition is especially diabetogenic.

 In the UK, diabetic retinopathy is the commonest cause of blindness between the ages of 30 and 64 years, comprising over 14% of all new blind registrations. The findings are similar in other developed countries. Although retinopathy is seldom seen within 5 years of the diagnosis of insulin-dependent diabetes, up to 80% of patients are affected after 15–20 years. About 15% of these patients have sight-threatening forms of retinopathy or maculopathy, and 1–2% will become blind unless adequately treated. There is no treatment which will guarantee maintenance of vision in patients with diabetic retinopathy. However, photocoagulation and vitrectomy have revolutionized treatment and vision can now be maintained in about 70% of patients who would otherwise have gone blind.

When diabetic nephropathy is established, the prognosis is seriously impaired. Proteinuria is present in about 10% of the diabetic clinic population, and its incidence increases with the duration of the diabetes. Proteinuria develops after about 15 years of diabetes and it is found in more than half the diabetics who have had diabetes for 30 years or more. Progressive deterioration is inevitable and, although the rate of progression is linear for each patient, the actual rate of decline varies considerably from one patient to another. Approximately three-quarters of patients are in terminal renal failure after 10 years of continuous proteinuria.

Coronary, cerebral and peripheral arterial disease represents the major cause of chronic ill health and premature death in both insulin-dependent and non-insulin-dependent diabetics in most westernized societies. The reasons for this enhanced susceptibility to atherosclerosis are uncertain. In part, it is due to the greater frequency of risk factors such as raised blood pressure and plasma lipids. However, the risk of arterial disease is amplified by other factors and the diabetic man is roughly twice as likely to die a cardiovascular death as the non-diabetic; the diabetic woman has an even higher risk. Raised arterial pressure is particulary damaging for the diabetic, greatly increasing the risk of cerebrovascular and coronary disease. Diabetic neuropathy is common in long-term diabetes. In women, the risk of diabetes increases with parity and those who give birth to large babies are likely to develop diabetes in later life.

Prevention

Many cases of diabetes mellitus could probably be prevented by suitable dieting and physical exercise, but the present evidence suggests the prevalence will rise as exercise disappears from our lives.

Screening for diabetes is unrealiable. The glucose-oxidase strip test is highly sensitive but it produces many false positive results. The copper-reduction tablet test is less sensitive and detects other reducing substances as well as glucose, but it is more specific in being able to identify negative specimens of urine correctly. Afer a standard 5 g oral glucose load, 30% in the Bedford study showed glycosuria but two-thirds of these were false positives, i.e. they were not hyperglycaemic. It is not known whether the detection of unsuspected diabetes and control of their blood sugar levels can greatly slow down the complications of diabetes — cataract, neuropathy, nephropathy and vascular disease. Nevertheless, some feel that the identification of early diabetes would be beneficial; the groups for which selective screening would be indicated are high parity women and the relatives of known cases. Although the incidence of diabetes is known to decrease with food shortages, there have been no intervention studies to show whether moderate dietary changes can reduce the incidence of diabetes in a community.

HYPERTHYROIDISM

Hyperthyroidism (thyrotoxicosis) results from the excess of circulating thyroid hormones, thyroxine and triiodothyronine. In the UK, 99% of cases are due to either Graves' disease (diffuse hyperplasia and hypertrophy of the thyroid gland) or Plummer's disease (hyperactive single or multiple nodules of the thyroid).

Epidemiology

It is a common disorder with a prevalence in adult women of about 2%. Males are affected less often and the female/male ratio is 5–10:1. Graves' disease occur at all ages but the incidence peaks at 20–40 years and toxic nodular goitre peaks between 40 and 70 years.

Prevention

There are no known preventive measures.

HYPOTHYROIDISM

The term 'hypothyroidism' denotes the slowing down of all body functions that results from a deficiency of circulating thyroid hormone. The term 'myxoedema' is usually applied to more severe forms of the disease in which deposition of mucous substances leads to the thickening of the skin and subcutaneous tissues.

Epidemiology

It is estimated that endemic goitre due to iodine deficiency affects about 200 million people worldwide. Other important causes of hypothyroidism are idiopathic atrophy of the thyroid gland, administration of antithyroid drugs, surgical removal of the thyroid, radiation and Hashimoto's disease. Areas with a high prevalence of endemic goitre are determined by certain geographical features, e.g. mountainous (the Alps and Himalayas), alluvial plains (the Great Lake basin of Canada and the USA) and areas where water supplies permeate through limestone (the Peak District of England, giving rise to the so-called 'Derbyshire neck'). The disease is more prevalent in women, with a female:male ratio of about 5:1. It occurs at all ages but the incidence peaks at 40–60 years.

Prevention

Dietary iodine deficiency is the major cause of endemic goitre and the disease is being slowly eradicated through iodination of foodstuffs or intramuscular injection of slow-release organic iodide compounds.

BREAST CANCER

Carcinoma of the breast, which accounts for 80% of breast tumours, has an extremely complex aetiology and epidemiology. All varieties of carcinoma arise from the epithelium of the duct system.

Epidemiology

Breast cancer is the most common malignancy in women in the Western world. Approximately 1 in every 13 women suffer from breast cancer during their lives. There are 21 000 registrations each year in England and Wales in women, representing a quarter of all female cancer registrations. The annual death toll of 12 000 women represents 20% of all female cancer deaths and 4% of all female deaths. In women it is the most common cause of death in the age group 35–54 years and the most common cause of cancer death in the age group 25–84 years. The incidence rises rapidly between 25 and 45 years, and thereafter more slowly. (*Fig. 11.1*).

In the UK, the incidence of breast cancer has risen steadily during the last 25 years, the increase being of the order of 1% per annum. Fatality rates have changed little.

The incidence of breast cancer increases with age except for a lull in middle life, the rate of increase being greatest before the menopause.

Breast cancer is most common in Northern Europe and North America and least commmon in Asia (including Japan) and Africa; intermediate rates are found in Southern Europe and South America. In all countries where the disease is common, the age-related increase in incidence is similar to that in Britain. However, in low-risk countries the incidence declines after the menopause. Premenopausal breast cancer shows much less international variation in incidence than the postmenopausal disease.

Jews are more likely to suffer from breast cancer and negroes less likely, although these differences are lessening over time. Migrant communities experience a slow change in breast cancer incidence.

In most countries, breast cancer is more common in the higher social classes. For example, in England, standardized registration ratios are 110 for non-manual classes and 82 for manual classes. But there is less variation in

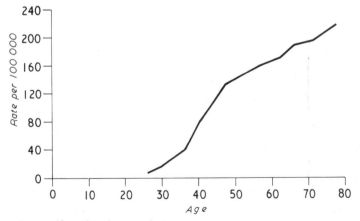

Fig. 11.1 Age-specific registration rates for breast cancer.

mortality, probably because of later presentation and poorer prognosis among the lower social classes.

The following risk factors have been examined.

1. Genetic — First-degree relatives have at least a two-fold risk of developing the disease, the risk being highest for premenopausal cases and those with bilaterial disease.
2. Childbearing — A large number of studies have established that early childbearing protects against breast cancer, the risk of which is three times greater in those bearing their first full-term infant at age 35 years or later than in those who have their first child before the age of 18 years. This is true in all communities and applies to both premenopausal and postmenopausal cancer. Nulliparous women appear to be at no greater risk than those who start childbearing in their thirties. Childbearing itself may represent a cancer risk in 'elderly' primigravidae. It now appears that high parity confers additional protection after account has been taken of the age at first pregnancy.
3. Lactation — It had long been thought that lactation conferred protection against breast cancer. A Chinese tribe, which characteristically fed from one breast only experienced less neoplasia on that side. However most of the apparent protection from breast feeding can be explained in terms of parity.
4. Hormonal factors — A number of epidemiological and clinical features suggest that hormone status is critical in the aetiology of breast cancer. These include the age distribution of cases, the rarity of the disease in men, the higher incidence in Klinefelter's syndrome, the response to hormone ablation, the relationship with parity, the protection conferred by oophorectomy and the carcinogenic effects of oestrone and other hormones in animals. Epidemiological observations fit the hypothesis that unopposed oestrogenic action increases the risk of breast cancer. Thus in addition to late childbearing, early menarche and late menopause are associated with an increased risk.

   In view of this, concern has arisen over the potential neoplastic hazards of oral contraceptives and postmenopausal hormone replacement. The latter probably doubles the risk of breast cancer; no clear evidence yet exists to incriminate oral contraceptives but it must be remembered that there is a latent period of 15 years or more.
5. Benign breast disease — The existence of fibrocystic disease of the breast is associated with a 2–4-fold increased risk of breast cancer. The two diseases share a number of important epidemiological features such as low parity, late menopause and high social class.
6. Diet — Animal studies have suggested that a high-fat diet increases the risk of breast cancer. National fat intake data correlate closely with the incidence of breast cancer but case–control studies have shown only a weak association.

7. Radiation — Atomic bomb survivors and patients exposed to high doses of therapeutic or diagnostic radiation have an increased risk of breast cancer. This may also apply to mammography. Data suggest that exposure during the second decade (when breast growth is maximal) is the most damaging.
8. Others — A viral aetiology in mice has been demonstrated but no evidence, epidemiological or otherwise, exists to implicate an infective aetiology in humans. A number of case–control studies have implicated the antihypersensitive agent reserpine in the aetiology of breast cancer but further research has failed to confirm these findings. Conflicting results have also been obtained in studies of the role of hair dyes.

To summarize, the most important established risk factors are genetic susceptibility, childbearing, hormonal status and benign breast disease. The most promising advances in our understanding of the aetiology and epidemiology of breast cancer are likely to be in the fields of diet and exogenous oestrogens.

Prevention

Primary prevention of such a complex disease will never be simple. However, there are good reasons to recommend a reduction in fat intake, to exercise caution in the use of therapeutic oestrogens, to avoid unnecessary radiation (especially during the teens) and to advise women who plan to have children that, if other considerations do not interfere, they should begin their family by the age of 25 years.

Most investment has been made into secondary prevention through the use of clinical examination and mammography to diagnose the disease at an early and curable stage. The first large-scale screening for breast cancer, conducted by the Health Insurance Plan of New York, at first showed a benefit (30% reduction in mortality at 10 years) only for women aged over 50 years. Other studies in the USA, Sweden and the Netherlands have confirmed the value of screening by mammography but there is still uncertainty about the optimal frequency. Screening of women aged 50–64 years at three-yearly intervals is being recommended in the UK.

Breast cancer in men

Breast cancer is rare in men. There are less than 200 new cases per annum in the UK. The incidence increases steadily with age. Male breast cancer is more common in Jews and rare in Japanese. The incidence is highest in Egypt where breast cancer accounts for 6% of male cancers. Raised oestrogen levels appear to confer an increased risk.

12

Disorders of the blood and haemopoietic system

IRON DEFICIENCY ANAEMIA

This is an anaemia brought about by inadequacy of body iron stores, characterized by progression from a normochromic normocytic to a hypochromic microcytic blood picture, which is responsive to treatment with iron and in which there is no other disease to explain the symptoms and blood picture. It may result from an inadequate intake of dietary iron, an inability to absorb the iron present in the diet or a persistent blood loss. These factors, alone or in combination, will eventually give rise to a hypochromic anaemia. In men, iron balance is fairly stable and a low haemoglobin will often indicate a serious disease such as cancer. In women, iron balance is precarious, and fairly severe anaemia can develop due to menstrual blood loss. Anaemia due to folate and B_{12} deficiency is rare and does not constitute a major problem in the Western world.

Epidemiology

After the first 10 years of life, mean haemoglobin levels are significantly higher in males than in females and the World Health Organization has defined anaemia as the occurrence of a haemoglobin level below 13 g/dl in men and 12 g/dl in adult non-pregnant women. But community surveys have shown that levels of circulating haemoglobin have a continuous distribution with a slight negative skewness and kurtosis. This makes the definition of anaemia by reference to a single level of haemologbin rather meaningless, implying a dichotomy of 'normal' and 'anaemic'.

Although iron deficiency anaemia occurs most frequently in developing countries, surveys in Western Europe have shown the wide prevalence of this condition. In England and Wales, the prevalence of haemoglobin levels of less than 13 g/dl in men is 6%, and of less than 12 g/dl in women 7%. In infancy, iron deficiency anaemia is twice as prevalent in the poorer areas of Britain as in middle-class areas.

138

In representative population samples of women, research has failed to demonstrate a significant correlation between haemoglobin level and the classic symptoms of anaemia. Similarly, there is no evidence to support the value of iron therapy for women with haemoglobin levels above 8 g/dl; the treatment of mild or moderate iron deficiency anaemia does not appear to lead to any detectable improvement in symptoms or 'fitness'.

In a population survey of iron deficiency anaemia, dysphagia and postcricoid web, no evidence was found that the syndrome of all three in the same person occurred any more often than would be expected from the chance association of the three unrelated conditions.

Prevention

Because iron balance is largely dependent on iron intake, attempts are made in some countries to reduce the prevalence of iron deficiency by the fortification of staple foodstuffs, such as bread, with iron. In the UK, where 40% of the iron in white bread has been added, about 25% of the iron intake is obtained from white bread and flour products. Nevertheless, there is as yet no convincing evidence of the preventive value of iron fortification of foodstuffs.

THE LEUKAEMIAS

The leukaemias involve the proliferation of lymphoid or of myeloid cells and, by tradition, 'acute' and 'chronic' forms of each are recognized. Each type includes well-defined subtypes with distinctive clinical patterns and responsiveness to treatment. Because leukaemia often affects young adults, its economic and emotional impact on family life is great.

Epidemiology

The overall incidence of leukaemia is fairly stable in the young but is increasing at older ages as a result of a rise in the incidence of chronic lymphocytic leukaemia (CLL). The four types of leukaemia together account for more than 3500 new cases a year in the UK with a slight excess of the myeloid type. Acute lymphocytic leukaemia (ALL) occurs mainly in children with a peak incidence at ages 2–8 years; there is another peak in the very old. ALL accounts for 85% of childhood leukaemias, most of the remainder being acute myeloid leukaemia (AML). There are approximately 600 new cases of ALL a year in the UK. AML (with 1500 new cases a year) is the most common type of adult leukaemia. Chronic leukaemias are rare in childhood, and CLL is particularly rare before 40 being usually a disease of advanced age. Overall, leukaemia occurs slightly more frequently in men than in women. The male/

female ratio for CLL is 2:1 (possibly reflecting occupational factors), and for AML 3:2.

One important known external aetiological factor is ionizing radiation. The earliest evidence of this came from cases arising soon after the discovery of X-rays; it was shown that leukaemia was particularly common among radiologists, although the excess risk has now decreased as safeguards in radiation practice have improved. The incidence of leukaemia was also high in radium dial painters who unwittingly ingested radium salts from their paint brushes. An increased incidence of leukaemia has been observed in a follow-up of men who received X-ray therapy for ankylosing spondylitis and in survivors of the nuclear explosions at Hiroshima and Nagasaki.

Retrospective studies have shown that *in-utero* exposure to X-ray appears to increase the risk of developing leukaemia in childhood. However, we cannot be certain that the association is a causal one. Exposure to ionizing radiation in high dosage increases the incidence of ALL and CML, but background levels of radiation are not now thought to have the same effect. Therapeutic exposure to radiation, alkylating agents or both increases the risk of AML. For example, about 5% of patients treated for Hodgkin's disease by both radiotherapy and chemotherapy who survive 5 years are likely to die of AML. Evidence that certain chemicals are leukaemogenic is strongest for benzene.

Human T-cell leukaemia/lymphoma virus (HTLV) is strongly associated with a particular histological subtype of lymphocytic leukaemia in Japan (adult T-cell leukaemia). This is suggestive of a viral aetiology for certain leukaemias.

Ethnic differences in the incidence of leukaemia at all ages show an increased incidence for white compared with black people. It occurs with greatly increased frequency in Down's syndrome (G trisomy) and probably in other varieties of non-disjunction. Among persons with Down's syndrome, leukaemia is 20 times more common than in the general population; all types of leukaemia are probably involved.

The leukaemias are not common causes of death; they account for only 2% of cancer deaths. The prognosis of ALL in children, especially those aged between 3 and 10 years, has changed dramatically in the last decade. There has been a steady improvement in the results of successive trials since 1970 and, in the group with the most favourable prognosis, about 80% are now curable.

Prevention

The two areas in which prevention may be successful are the control of exposure to man-made sources of ionizing radiation (used for diagnostic and therapeutic purposes) and to various chemicals with leukaemogenic potential.

THE LYMPHOMAS

There are two types: Hodgkin's disease (characterized by the presence of Reed–Sternberg giant cells) and non-Hodgkin's lymphoma.

Epidemiology

Hodgkin's disease is relatively uncommon; in Europeans the incidence is 3 per 100 000 for men and 1.8 per 100 000 for women.

There have been numerous reports of multiple occurrences of Hodgkin's disease within families. Siblings of the same sex have a risk double that of siblings of the opposite sex. There is a clear association between disease risk and sibship size.

Although there have been many reports of an association with occupational exposures to chemicals (such as benzene) and other substances, it is not yet known whether occupational factors increase the risk of disease.

Survival in Hodgkin's disease has undergone a dramatic change as a result of modern cancer therapy and the disease is now largely curable, especially in persons with Stage I and IIA disease (staged by laparotomy). However, treated Hodgkin's disease patients are at increased risk of developing other cancers.

The incidence of non-Hodgkin's lymphoma is twice that of Hodgkin's disease and it appears to be rising in some parts of the world. There is a slight male excess. Age-specific incidence shows a pre-adolescent peak and then a steady increase with age. In general, childhood Hodgkin's disease occurs with greater frequency in less developed countries and the young adult disease in developed Western countries. In the USA it is much less common in black people than in whites.

It would seem that radiation can induce the disease only after relatively heavy exposure (over 100 rads). The association between Epstein–Barr virus and Burkitt's lymphoma has stimulated efforts to link this and other viruses with non-Hodgkin's lymphoma. The discovery of HTLV has finally provided evidence for a long suspected viral aetiology of leukaemias and lymphomas. The virus is endemic in parts of Japan, the Caribbean, Central and South America and Africa and is associated with limited subtypes of NHL. Both congenital and acquired immune suppression appear to increase the risk of developing lymphoma.

Prevention

There are at present no known methods for the prevention of the lymphomas.

13

Abnormalities of growth and development

LOW BIRTHWEIGHT

This term is applied to babies who weigh 2500 g or less at birth.

Epidemiology

These babies constitute in Britain only 7% of the newborn, yet two-thirds of all perinatal deaths occur in this group. Low birthweight may be due either to shortening of the period of gestation, or to slowing of the rate of intrauterine growth, or to any combination of the two. Two-thirds of these births are truly premature, i.e. the babies are born before 37 completed weeks from the first day of the mother's last menstrual period. In most cases, the cause of the early onset of labour is unknown. The babies' problems are those of immaturity and the major cause of death is hyaline membrane disease which occurs with increasing frequency and severity at decreasing gestational ages. The other group of low birthweight babies are those who are light for the gestational age at which they are born, either because of poor growth potential (including fetal malformation and intrauterine infection such as rubella) or a growth-restricting intrauterine environment. In the latter group, maternal factors have an important influence on fetal growth, especially poor socioeconomic status. The problems occurring in light-for-dates babies are intrauterine hypoxia, birth asphyxia and symptomatic hypoglycaemia.

In the first 2 years of life, low birthweight babies are more liable to colds and coughs and to have an excess of hospital admissions for lower respiratory infections. Physical growth, intelligence, neurological status and behavioural and learning ability are all adversely affected in babies who are below the tenth centile of weight for gestation. Light-for-dates babies fare significantly worse than the pre-term. The evidence to-date shows that babies born after a shortened gestation, although at a disadvantage, can be expected to develop significantly better than babies whose intrauterine growth has been slowed to a comparable degree, provided they receive an adequate standard of nutrition and general care during the period which ought to have been spent in the uterus.

There is evidence that intensive neonatal care (introduced in the 1960s) has exerted an appreciable effect on the early mortality of low birthweight infants. However, concern has been expressed that the increase in survival may have been achieved at the expense of an increase in the proportion of those left with severe physical and mental handicaps. The findings of epidemiological studies are encouraging in that there has been, in many countries, a decrease in the prevalence of spastic diplegia — a condition that has, in the past, been most often associated with pre-term births.

The relationships between low birthweight and a number of social and biological factors are shown in *Table 13.1*. The proportion of low birthweight births (1) increases with descent in the social scale; (2) shows a U-shaped pattern for maternal age and for parity (which are highly correlated); (3) is higher among illegitimate births than among legitimate; and (4) is high

Table 13.1 Low birthweight according to social and biological factors; England and Wales, 1984

Factors	Percentage of live births weighing less than 2500 g
All live births	6.7
Social class (legitimate births):	
I	5.6
II	5.7
III non-manual	6.2
III manual	7.0
IV	8.3
V	8.1
Age:	
Under 20	8.7
20–24	7.1
25–29	6.1
30–34	7.1
35 +	7.2
Parity: (legitimate)	
0	7.5
1	5.0
2	5.4
3+	6.9
Legitimacy:	
Illegitimate	9.0
Legitimate	6.2
Mother's place of birth:	
United Kingdom	6.5
Irish Republic	5.8
India and Bangladesh	10.1
Africa	11.0
West Indies	6.7
Pakistan	8.9

among births to mothers born in India and Bangladesh, Africa or Pakistan.

Mean birthweight is reduced in babies born to mothers who are short (less than 1.6 m (5'2") or who smoke (a mean reduction of 170 g has been reported). In one study, maternal height was shown to be responsible for 50% of the variance in birthweight.

Prevention

The incidence of low birthweight might be expected to fall as social and economic conditions improve — but it has not yet done so. Health education on the harmful effects of smoking is clearly an important preventive measure in reducing the number of light-for-dates babies. The incidence of pre-term birth can also be influenced to some extent by obstetric care, e.g. cervical cerclage, early diagnosis of multiple pregnancy and the suppression of premature labour.

CONGENITAL MALFORMATIONS

A congenital malformation is a macroscopic abnormality of structure attributed to faulty development and present at birth.

Epidemiology

Since the causes of most malformations are unknown, some arbitrary classification has to be devised and this is usually by anatomical system. In determining the prevalence of these conditions at birth, the notification of birth form is a valuable source of information. However, some defects may not be apparent at birth and so reasonable completeness of ascertainment can be assumed only when all possible sources of information have been tapped. These include registrations of stillbirth and death, notifications from clinicians, health visitors and pathologists, registers of handicapped children and hospital discharge records. In Britain, there is a monitoring scheme in which malformations detected within 7 days of birth are reported to the District Medical Officer on a voluntary basis. These notifications are forwarded to the Office of Population Censuses and Surveys for analysis.

Population surveys have shown that in Britain between 2 and 4% of infants are malformed at birth, the most common defects being those of the central nervous system (mainly anencephaly and spina bifida cystica) and of the heart and great vessels (*Table 13.2*). Major malformations resulting in chronic handicap or necessitating surgery are present in about 2% of liveborn infants. The birth prevalence of some malformations is very different from the true incidence (i.e. the proportion of embryos in which they are laid down). This is because many malformed embryos abort spontaneously. Some typical esti-

Table 13.2 The prevalence at birth of selected malformations in Britain

Type of malformation	Prevalence per 1000 total births
Anencephaly	1.4–4.2*
Spina bifida aperta (without anencephaly)	1.5–4.5*
Abnormalities of the heart and great vessels	6.9
Cleft lip and/or palate	2.0
Pyloric stenosis	2.2
Dislocation of the hip(s)	0.9
Down's syndrome	1.2

*The rates are for London (low) and Belfast (high) in the 1960s

mates of the miscarriage rate in the UK are: anencephaly 73%, spina bifida 29%, congenital anomalies of the heart and great vessels 71% and Down's syndrome 65%.

Congenital malformations are responsible for one in five perinatal and infant deaths. Fatality rates vary with the nature and extent of the malformation. All anencephalic babies die. Active surgical treatment of spina bifida has increased survival from 20% to around 60% of liveborn cases. Overall case-fatality is around 30% in congenital heart lesions. Survival in Down's syndrome has increased enormously with the control of infectious disease in the community.

There is good evidence that environmental influences are involved since the prevalence rates of various defects show geographical, secular and seasonal fluctuations and social class, maternal age and parity differences. In addition, the concordance rate for identical twins is well below 100% for most malformations, although higher than for fraternal twins of like sex. Discordance in identical twin pairs is almost the rule in some malformations, for example anencephaly.

While some of the marked international differences in the incidence of congenital malformations (such as the low rate of neural tube defects in negro populations and in Japan) are likely to be largely genetic in origin, the geographical variations within the British Isles in malformation incidence remain unexplained. Most prominent among these are the high incidence of anencephaly in Northern Ireland, and of anencephaly and spina bifida in South Wales.

Many congenital malformations are more common among first births, but anencephaly and spina bifida show a U-shaped trend with parity. Two conditions are known to be age-dependent: Down's syndrome, in which trisomy 21 (but not translocation) is related to maternal age (*Fig. 13.1*) and achondroplasia, which increases with paternal age. The incidence of most congenital defects is higher among male infants than among female; a small number, for example anencephaly and congenital dislocation of the hip, show a female preponderance.

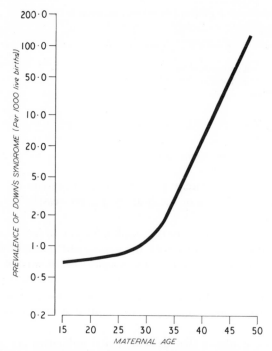

Fig. 13.1 Down's syndrome: the prevalence at birth in relation to maternal age.

Several studies have shown that neural tube defects have a higher prevalence among poorer families, the social class difference being greatest in anencephaly. Dietary deficiencies (e.g. of vitamins) may play an important part in producing this class pattern.

Seasonal variations in incidence have been reported for some malformations, for example an excess among winter births for anencephaly (although much of this seasonal pattern has now disappeared) and for congenital dislocation of the hip.

Many enquiries have been made into teratogenic influences in pregnancy. Evidence from retrospective studies must be interpreted with caution for two reasons: (1) mothers of malformed babies may look for explanations for their misfortune and so remember, or even imagine, past events that mothers of normal children are more likely to forget; and (2) even if malformations are found to be more common in those exposed to a putative teratogen, there is still the possibility that the real cause of the increase is not this factor but something else that tends to affect the same people. The possibility of mothers' memories being influenced by the birth of a malformed child can be circumvented by undertaking a prospective study.

Around 20% of all recognized pregnancies and 50% of all conceptions end in fetal death. At least half of all conceptions aborted have anatomical and/or chromosmal abnormalities which, in the majority of cases, are incompatible with survival. Women who have given birth to children with malformations of the central nervous system have a raised miscarriage rate among earlier pregnancies; in one study it was found that in these mothers more than 40% of all known pregnancies ended in either miscarriage or the birth of a child with a congenital defect. Studies of other pregnancy factors, such as illnesses and drugs have not been very fruitful with the exception of a small number of uncommon conditions such as the embryopathy due to rubella (*see* Chapter 2) and thalidomide. It now seems likely that, although environmental influences are undoubtedly important, they will prove to be much more subtle and much less accessible to control than was at one time hoped.

Prevention

The association of neural tube defects with social class suggests that improvements in socio-economic conditions should lead to a reduction in these malformations. A reduction in the number of high parity births will have a similar effect. The clinical measures available for the prevention of congenital malformations are:

1. Genetic counselling where a previous child has been affected or where there is a strong family history.
2. Rubella immunization of schoolgirls at 10–13 years.
3. Antenatal diagnosis of chromosomal abnormalities and neural tube defects, followed by termination of pregnancy.
4. The avoidance, as far as practicable, of drugs in the first trimester of pregnancy.
5. The maintenance of an adequate diet (including vitamins) in the periconceptional period and early months of pregnancy.

MENTAL HANDICAP

It is customary to make a division between severely mentally handicapped people, who may be defined as having IQs of below 50, and mildly handicapped persons who have IQs in the 50–70 range. The majority of mildly handicapped individuals are free of clinical indications of nervous system damage or defect. Severely handicapped individuals nearly always suffer some clearly demonstrable form of impairment which, in a significant number of cases, gives rise to physical disabilities such as epilepsy, spasticity, blindness and hearing defects. Overall, about one severely mentally handicapped person in three has a sensory or motor disability. The term 'mental handicap' is not usually applied to people who become mentally impaired in later life due to, for instance, road accidents, strokes or premature dementia.

Epidemiology

Although there is estimated to be more than one and a quarter million people in the UK with an IQ of less than 70, the number of people who have at some stage in their lives come to the notice of service-providing authorities as being mildly mentally handicapped or educationally subnormal (the 'administrative prevalence') is much lower, probably in the order of 400 000. In addition there are approximately 160 000 severely mentally handicapped people in the UK, 60 000 of whom are children.

Surveys have shown that between 2 and 3% of people in the UK have IQs below 70. Of these, just over 1 in 10 is severely affected. The prevalence of severe handicap at age seven is about 4 per 1000. Only about 5% of severely mentally handicapped children can achieve social and economic independence in adult life.

Since 1968 there has been a fall in the number of residents in mental handicap hospitals but this is because more are now living in local authority homes. Overall, the number in residential care has increased and this is partly because of longer survival. Although the prevalence of Down's syndrome has increased owing to greater survival, that of severe mental handicap overall has not. This implies a major reduction in some forms of handicapping event (such as pre- or post-natal damage associated with infection).

While there is no significant social class variation in the incidence and prevalence of severe mental handicap, the prevalence of mild handicap is roughly nine times greater among the children of unskilled manual workers than among those in non-manual occupations. This is a strong indication of selective environmental influences. Studies of mild handicap have revealed a consistent pattern of material deprivation, poor housing and the substandard educational opportunities linked to other factors such as large family size and family instability. In addition, it appears that sub-clinical physical defects and inadequate nutrition are particularly likely to influence adversely the physical and mental development of children in this group. While the available evidence does not support the concept of an inbred stable social class with an inferior genetic endowment, there is some evidence indicating a tendency towards downwards social drift among the parents of a proportion of mildly handicapped children.

There is no evidence that complications of delivery or birth injury are important causes of severe mental subnormality but it has been shown that, for both the severely and educationally subnormal groups, there is an excess of babies of low birthweight as compared with groups of mentally normal children. About 40% of all severe mental handicap is associated with specific genetic or chromosomal abnormalities, mainly Down's syndrome, which accounts for a quarter to a third of cases.

Prevention

Since adverse social and environmental conditions are responsible for the poor mental performance of many children, there is need for a degree of positive discrimination in the allocation of relevant health and social resources to localities with large proportions of disadvantaged families; and for the establishment of closer links between schools, day nurseries, day centres, relevant health services and voluntary organizations.

Measures to prevent severe mental handicap are given under the sections on low birthweight and congenital malformations. They include rubella immunization, improvement in perinatal care and the antenatal diagnosis of such conditions as Down's syndrome, spina bifida and Tay Sachs' disease, followed by termination of pregnancy.

SUDDEN INFANT DEATH SYNDROME

This has been defined as, 'the sudden death of any infant or young child, which is unexpected by history, and in which a thorough postmortem examination fails to demonstrate an adequate cause of death'.

Epidemiology

About half the post-neonatal deaths in the UK occur at home as unexpected 'cot deaths'. At autopsy, there is evidence of a definite disease state in a third of cases; this may be a severe acute disease (such as meningitis, acute obstructive tracheobronchitis, or gastroenteritis with hypernatraemia) or a chronic condition (such as a congenital malformation). In a third, there are no features of acute disease at autopsy and in a further third a lesion that would be expected to cause only minor illness. These last two groups together constitute what is usually referred to as the sudden infant death syndrome (SIDS). The problems with the use of the term SIDS are that (1) it encourages the view that it is a clinical entity with a single cause, and (2) it is dependent on the amount and quality of the information available.

The incidence of 'cot deaths' in the UK is around 2 per 1000 live births. The peak age incidence of SIDS occurs at 12–16 weeks and it is uncommon after 9 months. The male:female ratio is 1.5:1. The incidence of these deaths is highest in socially deprived families characterized by young maternal age, low parental intelligence, poor maternal efficiency and a multiplicity of problems including poor housing, illegitimacy, cohabitation or a tense marital situation. In this group, too, there is evidence of failure by the parents to recognize serious illness in their baby. A study of the obstetric and perinatal histories of babies dying of SIDS has shown that the most powerful criterion for identifying high-risk children is failure of the mother to bring the baby to the first follow-up clinic after discharge from hospital.

The seasonal incidence (an excess in January and March in the UK) and social class pattern favour an infective cause for SIDS. Overlaying, suffocation from bedclothes or a soft pillow, and inhalation of regurgitated milk are now believed to be uncommon causes. All the common respiratory pathogens have been isolated in SIDS and it has been suggested that a high proportion of these deaths is due to a fulminating infection of the lower respiratory tract. Attempts at virus isolation have been disappointing and there is no evidence that overwhelming virus infection is a common feature in SIDS.

Many other causes have been suggested for these unexplained deaths, including nasal obstruction in those infants who are unable to substitute oral breathing if the nose is obstructed, and hypoglycaemia due to nocturnal fasting or to an excess of protein in the feeds. But we are probably not considering a single disease entity, and all that can be said at present is that the characteristic age range suggests that, while passing through a period of increased physiological vulnerability, some critical combination of intrinsic and extrinsic factors proves lethal.

Prevention

Evidence from Sheffield suggests that, by identifying babies 'at risk' and providing additional health visiting to these families, the incidence of SIDS can be reduced. The education of parents in the recognition of signs of illness in their baby is an important aspect of health visiting. After one SIDS in a family, the use of an apnoea alarm for subsequent babies will provide reassurance for the parents and may help to prevent a further death.

PROTEIN ENERGY MALNUTRITION

The World Health Organization has defined protein energy malnutrition as 'a range of pathological conditions arising from coincident lack, in varying proportions, of protein and calories, occurring most frequently in infants and young children and commonly associated with infections'. Mortality is usually due to infection.

Epidemiology

Protein energy malnutrition (PEM) of young children is without doubt the most important form of malnutrition in the world. The term encompasses a spectrum of syndromes ranging from simple growth failure alone to pure and mixed syndromes of marasmus, kwashiorkor, and even pellagra. This is due to the fact that diets vary enormously from region to region and also have seasonal fluctuations. Local factors — such as excessive heat or cold, drought or floods, tropical disease, overcrowding and poor sanitation — can modify or precipitate the presentation of PEM.

The clinical presentation of PEM varies with the degree and duration of protein and energy depletion, the age of the individual and the modifications produced by associated vitamin, mineral and trace element deficiencies. The well-known syndromes of marasmus and kwashiorkor are not as common as the mild form of PEM which may present with growth failure only.

In order to carry out prevalence studies in the community, the basic data should include age, weight, height, presence of oedema and additional signs of kwashiorkor, hepatomegaly, dermatosis, hair changes and evidence of associated deficiencies such as xerophthalmia and anaemia. The methodology and criteria vary considerably between studies but it has been estimated that about 100 million children throughout the world are suffering from moderate or severe PEM at any one time. Data based on hospitals or clinics give no idea of the true incidence in a community. Mortality rates in children, especially under the age of 5 years, are related to malnutrition and may be used as an indirect means of assessing the community's nutritional status.

It would seem that marasmus emerged on a large scale with the overcrowding and bad hygiene of rapidly growing cities, and that kwashiorkor resulted from the breakdown of tribal customs in the rural areas which previously ensured for the young child its full complement of breast feeding. Urban living is only inimical to the child's nutrition when poor sanitation and overcrowding lead to gastroenteritis and other debilitating conditions, and when the protective influence of breast feeding is abandoned under economic and cultural pressures. There is some evidence of a worldwide increase of marasmus and a decrease of kwashiorkor.

In developed countries there is a high prevalence of protein calorie malnutrition among patients in hospital (as many as 50% of surgical patients in one study). Some are admitted with an illness that has caused the problem; others develop nutritional problems while undergoing treatment. Major nutritional disorders undoubtedly prejudice recovery from surgical operations.

Prevention

The time and adequacy of weaning are crucial determinants of the nutrition of the young child in developing countries. Increase in food production is not necessarily the answer to the problem since severe PEM frequently occurs in the absence of overall food shortage but will accompany maldistribution of food within the family.

The important relationship between nutrition and infections needs to be kept in mind when nutrition programmes are being considered. It would be illogical to plan for improved diets for poor children without at the same time paying attention to the control of infectious diseases and the need for good health care for the poor.

The cause of malnutrition is frequently complex and there are often many interrelated causative factors involving both the human host and his environment. Intervention will be aimed at one or more, often several, of these underlying determinants. The control of PEM usually requires a variety of intervention activities conducted by health workers and many others from disciplines such as agriculture, education and community development.

OBESITY

An overweight person has a body weight above the desirable level, i.e. the weight at which greatest longevity can be expected. A desirable weight is usually calculated in relation to height, or height and build, often using tables devised by life insurance companies. An obese person has an abnormally high percentage of body fat with a consequent increase in morbidity.

Epidemiology

Excess fat accumulates because of imbalance between ingested food energy and energy expended. The nature of the regulatory mechanisms which maintain a relatively constant body weight is unknown but they can fail in a number of circumstances including a high fat diet, marked physical inactivity and genetically transmitted forms of obesity.

The body mass index (W/H^2 where W is weight in kilograms and H is height in metres) has the best correlation with body fat. The skinfold thickness has also been used to estimate obesity. Data from a variety of studies indicate that in both the UK and USA, about 1 adult in 10 is clinically obese. The distribution of obese males peaks at 40–55 years of age, compared with 50–60 years in females, but in most populations there are more obese females than males in each age group.

There is strong evidence pointing to a greater prevalence of obesity in the lower socioeconomic groups in highly industrialized countries. It seems that this begins early and is related to diet. In Kent, it was shown that children in the poorer classes had lower total nutrient intake than children in the higher social classes, but they consumed amounts of carbohydrate and added sugar equal to those of the higher social class children, so that the quality of the lower class diet was worse. The higher prevalence of obesity in the lower social classes applies only in countries where calorie supply is adequate at all income levels. In developing countries, obesity is more prevalent among the more privileged sections of society.

Life insurance statistics show that excess weight is associated with a significant increase in mortality when the body mass index (BMI) is above 30.

(This is the lower limit in obesity; the acceptable range is below 25, and the BMI in the grossly obese is 40 and above.) A study in Framingham involving 5000 people showed that increased relative weight was associated with a significant increase in sudden death and angina pectoris, but not with myocardial infarction. However, if other risk factors such as hypertension and high serum cholesterol levels are considered, obesity of itself loses significance. Although measurements of blood pressure are often overestimated if the arm is very fat, there is a genuine correlation between obesity and blood pressure.

Prevention

Careful attention to calorie intake and a regular programme of physical activity will prevent an increase in body fat with age. Obesity should be included in all screening programmes, at whatever age.

High blood pressure can be reduced in 50% of obese patients by weight loss. Impaired glucose tolerance and hyperinsulinaemia may also be reversed by weight loss, as may the detrimental effect of obesity in non-insulin-dependent diabetes mellitus.

14

Injuries

ACCIDENTAL INJURIES

The World Health Organization has defined an accident as 'an un-predetermined event resulting in a recognisable injury'. In Western Europe since the Second World War there has been a reversal of the roles of infectious disease and injury as causes of death, so that deaths from infection are now less than one-fifth of those due to injury. Both domestic and road traffic accident deaths have risen during this period but the main change has been a reduction in mortality from infection. Accidents are the leading cause of death and injury in persons age 1–40 years. They are exceeded only by cancer and ischaemic heart disease as a cause of loss of years of working life.

Although the injuries from different types of accident are often clinically similar, from the point of view of causation and prevention we need to classify accidents by the circumstances in which they occur. Most accidental injuries are related to domestic life (at least 40% in Britain), transport (another 40%) or occupation (4%). The rise in the total number of accidental deaths has been due to increases in domestic and transport accidents, whereas occupational deaths have tended to decrease.

The total accidental death rate in males has a peak in the twenties; from 50 years onwards it increases rapidly to a maximum in old age. Domestic accidents predominate in the preschool period; from about 10 to 15 years road traffic accidents are the main determinant of the total rate and thereafter domestic accidents again predominate. In childhood and early adult life, females follow the same pattern although with a much less prominent peak for road traffic accidents. The death rate for domestic accidents after 50 years, however, is much higher; it represents an even greater preponderance of cases, since females of 50 years of age and over outnumber males by one-third.

Injuries not causing death are much more numerous but there is no system of recording that applies equally to all types and circumstances of accident.

Domestic accidents

In the UK more than 6500 people die each year as a result of accidents at home and at play. The groups most at risk are children and elderly people.

The most common domestic accidents are falls, accounting for just over half of all deaths from accidents in the home. Burns and scalds are next in frequency but they are responsible for only 10% of home accidents; they are, however, the commonest type of accident in children.

Although much less frequent than previously, deaths from suffocation and respiratory obstruction by foreign bodies are still prominent in infants. Falls from furniture, scalds from falling into or overturning hot liquids and injuries from sharp objects affects both sexes about equally in preschool years. It is the children in the age group 1–4 years that are mainly at risk of accidental poisoning due to medicinal and household products. There is a pronounced social class gradient in childhood accidents with children in social class V having a mortality rate for falls, burning and drowning ten times the rate in class I.

At ages over 65 years, deaths in females (mainly due to femoral neck fractures) outnumber those in males by 60%, deaths of elderly females due to falls accounting for 40% of all domestic accident fatalities. A number of factors have been found to be associated with falls in the elderly. These include a history of stroke or heart disease, vertigo, sudden loss of consciousness, defects of vision, drugs (including alcohol) and environmental hazards such as loose carpeting, slippery floors or trailing wires. Deaths from accidental poisoning due to domestic gas (characteristically in elderly people with anosmia) have fallen dramatically with the change from coal gas to natural (North Sea) gas.

Transport accidents

Each year in Britain 100 000 people are admitted to hospital having been injured on the road; 80 000 are seriously injured. From a few hundred at the beginning of the century, the number of deaths in Britain from this cause each year is now over 7000. In the USA it is 46 000 and in West Germany (which has a population similar to that of Britain and a similar number of vehicles) 15 000.

The risk of a fatal accident is 30 times greater for motor cyclists (who suffer one-eighth of fatal accidents) than for car drivers. Pedal cyclists occupy an intermediate position (12 times the risk for car drivers). Accidents are more common in men than in women, and in younger drivers and motor cyclists. Age-specific death rates are shown in *Figure 14.1*. Deaths among pedestrians are mainly in the very young and the aged.

Head injuries and multiple fractures are the commonest causes of death

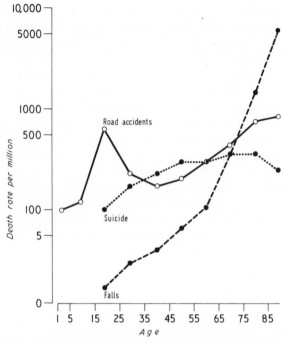

Fig. 14.1 Age-specific death rates for road transport accidents, falls and suicide in England and Wales.

from road accidents. Road traffic accidents account for about half the adult head injuries admitted to hospital. The incidence of severe head injuries reached a peak in the mid-1960s but has since declined, partly due to fewer motor cyclists and to the compulsory use of crash helmets. The case fatality in severe head injury is around 40% and, of these deaths, 40% occur before the patient reaches hospital and another 20% in the accident and emergency department. Twenty per cent of survivors have a residual disability due to brain damage.

The consumption of alcohol increases the risk of road traffic accidents, and the blood alcohol level is above the legal limit in one-third of drivers killed; not only does this affect drivers but a high proportion of pedestrians injured in road accidents are also found to have been drinking to excess. Since 1983, there has been reduction in deaths of drivers and front-seat passengers as a result of the compulsory wearing of seat-belts.

Industrial accidents

There are between 400 000 and 500 000 accidents at work each year in Britain, causing the loss of around 20 million working days. The nonmanufacturing industries have the highest accident rates; these include occupations such as coalmining and fishing. The incidence of industrial accidents is high in the teens and early twenties (probably because of lack of experience), declines in the third and fourth decades and then rises slightly until retirement is reached.

Accidents reach a peak when the work rate is fastest and they increase when a shift is lengthened. Rates are lower when there are good working relationships accompanied by good communications.

Each year in Britian there are about 1000 fatal industrial accidents. About two-fifths occur in factories, almost as many in construction work and one-third in mining. The main causes are falls and falling objects, which between them account for more than half the deaths. Falls are particularly prominent in building construction and in factories. There is a high rate of fatal accidents in older workers.

Prevention

Methods of prevention of domestic accidents follow from a knowledge of their causes. Improved housing and education in child care, increased awareness of the risks to children of burning accidents and drowning, and the use of practical methods of prevention of burns (such as fireguards) are clearly all important. The use of flame-resistant textiles for children's clothing and a sustained campaign about the danger of fireworks are both achieving success. Accidental poisoning can be greatly reduced by better packaging of drugs.

The prevention of road accidents is largely a question of devising and enforcing appropriate rules of behaviour such as speed limits, the wearing of seat belts and restricting alcohol intake. The introduction of breath tests in 1968 led to a significant reduction in injuries. Experiments have confirmed the benefits of improved street lighting at night in reducing accident rates and of improved vehicle design in reducing serious injuries.

Prevention of industrial accidents has received much attention from government, industry and voluntary organizations. Automation tends to achieve greater safety as well as greater efficiency. The introduction of low voltage power supplies, shielding of machinery and the use of protective clothing backed by educational campaigns are all helping to control the incidence of serious industrial injuries.

NON-ACCIDENTAL INJURIES

In 1946 Caffey, a paediatric radiologist, drew attention to the association between subdural haematomas and fractures of the long bones in young children. Gradually it was accepted that these and other injuries could be inflicted by parents and that non-accidental injury to children was by no means a rare occurrence.

The injuries are diverse, including bruises and lacerations, fractures of the skull, clavicles, ribs or long bones, burns, scalds and cerebral damage. Subdural effusion and retinal haemorrhages are probably caused by vigorous shaking. Deliberate poisoning is another form of child abuse.

Epidemiology

The estimated incidence in the USA is not less than 6 per thousand live births and it is believed to be responsible for about 25% of all fractures in children under the age of 2 years. In the UK the estimated incidence is around 4500 per annum with a fatality rate of not less than 3%.

Many of the affected children also show evidence of previous neglect, maltreatment and emotional deprivation which is reflected in poor nutrition and stunted growth. A case–control study has shown that the majority of the mothers show evidence of emotional immaturity and many of them have a history of recurrent depression. A psychopathic personality has been diagnosed in one-third of the fathers and almost as many have a criminal record. Several studies have shown that battered children come from all social classes but in the case–control study mentioned above the parents were predominantly from social classes IV and V.

Most investigators agree that the parents tend to come from unhappy backgrounds and were possibly battered children themselves. There is a tendency for battering parents to be young, often still in their teens. The families are frequently isolated both physically and emotionally with few contacts outside the nuclear family. In an American study, some 10% of the mothers were single, 20% were alone as a result of separation, divorce, desertion or widowhood and in 12% of cases the biological mother was not living at home. There is an increased risk of a subsequent child being similarly maltreated.

One study has identified six factors as significant — abnormal pregnancy, abnormal labour or delivery, neonatal separation, some other separation in the first 6 months of life, illness of the child in the first year of life and illness of the mother in the first year of the child's life.

In a careful follow-up of abused children who were examined 3 years later, more than half were impaired neurologically and one-third of these were severely mentally retarded. Even where they do not have identifiable brain damage or mental handicap, they still show significant learning failure at school and impaired emotional development.

Prevention

The first step towards prevention is the early recognition of 'at risk' families. Opportunities already exist during attendance at antenatal clinics, in maternity units and during follow-up visits by nurses and health visitors, and during visits of mothers and infants or toddlers to child health clinics. This should be followed by discussion of anxieties and anticipation of problems which might require guidance. At the time of delivery, doctors and nurses should be aware of the importance of promoting the bonding process, especially by avoiding physical separation of mother and baby.

Vigilance is also needed by general practitioners, especially when a harassed mother seems to be at the end of her tether with a difficult infant or young child or makes frequent vague complaints and seems apathetic. The staff of accident and emergency departments need training in the recognition not only of non-accidental injuries but also of children at risk. Of importance, too, are the avoidance of unwanted pregnancies by the provision of adequate family planning services, careful surveillance of the siblings of battered children and realistic preparation for parenthood as part of the school curriculum. Registers of battered children can be helpful in confirming the doctor or social worker's suspicion that an injury may be non-accidental.

15

Psychiatric disorders

Between a quarter and a third of all illnesses treated by general practitioners in Britain are diagnosable as mental disorders, and about 15% of the adult population present to their general practitioners with a mental disorder in a year. In Britain 30 million working days are lost each year as a result of mental illness.

Psychiatric disorders are the leading cause of hospital admission in Britain. The Mental Health Enquiry in England and Wales, which is concerned with all admissions to psychiatric units from 1964 onwards, has shown that there are about four admissions per 1000 population. Psychiatric case registers indicate that about 1% of the population has a new episode of outpatient or inpatient care each year. About 40% of hospital beds in the UK are occupied by patients suffering from mental illness. There has been a gratifying increase in the number of patients who seek hospital treatment on an informal basis, while the number of compulsory patients has been showing a steady decline. This has been accompanied by a considerable increase in the discharge rate as a result of early and improved methods of treatment, but there is still a high re-admission rate. A survey of mental illness in general practice has suggested that there may be twice as many mentally disabled persons in the community as in mental hospitals.

A survey of London practices revealed that only 1 in 4 major psychoses and 1 in 20 of all psychiatric cases were referred for specialist treatment during the survey year. Psychotic patients and patients with personality disorders tend to be referred to the specialist, leaving the general practitioner with mainly the cases of neurosis.

The two main problems inherent in psychiatric epidemiology are:

1. The difficulty in defining the conditions to be studied.
2. The development of field techniques capable of allowing their full identification in a given population.

Using records going back as far as 1840, workers in Massachusetts compared the nineteenth century and contemporary age-specific first admission rates for psychoses. They showed that for ages under 50, admission rates were just as high during the last half of the nineteenth century as they are now. There has, however, been a very marked increase in admission rates in the older age groups — an increase which appears to be due mainly to the increased tendency to hospitalize people suffering from mental illness in old age. They concluded that there has been no long-term increase in the incidence of the psychoses in early and middle life, and that social trends probably have little influence on the incidence of psychosis. The UK experienced a doubling of the general practitioner consultation rates for mental disorder between the First and Second National Morbidity Studies of 1951 and 1971. This rise in the demand for care may be due to a real change in the prevalence of mental disorder or a change in attitudes on the part of patients.

The maximum incidence of mental disorder in males lies between the ages of 30 and 40 and in females between 25 and 35. After these ages there is a fall, followed by an increase at the involutional period and in old age. The increasing age of the population has been associated with an increase in the depressive reactions and in the organic, degenerative mental disorders of later life. Two-thirds of the patients aged 65 and over in the mental hospitals in Britain are women, no doubt mainly because women live longer than men.

We know comparatively little about the distribution of mental illness in Britain and the USA. We know less about these conditions in most other countries and very litte indeed about any country outside the Western civilization.

NEUROSES

Neuroses are psychiatric disorders in which the personality remains intact, contact with reality is preserved and symptoms are subjective, persistent and troublesome. The neurotic is preoccupied with his symptoms, often morose and invariably frustrated and querulous. Symptoms include low energy, a feeling of malaise, inability to cope, insomnia and feelings of anxiety and tension.

Epidemiology

Neuroses are the most common psychiatric disorders but accurate estimates of the prevalence are difficult to obtain because the diagnosis is often imprecise. Many illnesses are diagnosed as neurotic by general practitioners when they are in fact affective psychoses. About half of all psychiatric outpatients appear to suffer from neuroses; so also do many of those who attend surgical and medical clinics at general hospitals.

Neurotic illness is most prevalent among middle-aged women. The aspects of the life of suburban areas of our large cities which may be inimical to mental health and productive of neurosis are boredom, anxiety (about money, housing and having another baby) and false values due to the decline of religious faith and its replacement by the values of the advertisers. Other social factors are the effects of rehousing in producing family and social dislocation and the loneliness of life on housing estates where each family tends to keep to itself. Frequently there is a morbid family environment such as may be produced by maternal anxiety, parental quarrelling or some other form of broken home. These are the predisposing factors. The immediate factors include any source of dissatisfaction or exposure to some overwhelming stress.

In the genesis of an anxiety neurosis there is commonly an inherited predisposition. One-fifth of the parents of patients with anxiety states have a similar disorder.

Prevention

There are no specific preventive measures.

DEPRESSION

This is a persistent flattening of mood accompanied by a poor self-image and biological features such as anorexia, weight loss, slowing of thoughts and loss of libido.

Epidemiology

Questionnaires have been designed for use in population surveys but estimates of the prevalence of depression show a three-fold variation. In Britain, it appears to be more common in urban than in rural areas. Both hospital admission rates and community studies indicate a female:male ratio of about 2:1. It is more prevalent among separated and divorced individuals, but the relationship is not clear.

Psychosocial factors involved include major life events such as loss by death or separation in the presence of certain risk factors such as unemployment, early loss of the mother or a large number of children.

Prevention

There are no known preventive measures.

SCHIZOPHRENIA

The diagnosis of schizophrenia is made on the grounds of whether or not 'first rank symptoms' are present. These include auditory hallucinations, passivity experiences and primary delusions. Passivity experiences are thoughts, emotions, impulses or actions experienced by the individual as if under external alien control; primary delusions often commence with a sense of revelation, the subject believing he or she has suddenly understood a previously hidden truth.

Epidemiology

Admission rates to mental hospitals in England indicate a lifetime incidence rate for schizophrenia between 0.8 and 0.9%. There are currently some 6000 new cases diagnosed in the UK annually and it is believed that there are over 300 000 people in Britain today who have had at some time a condition diagnosed as schizophrenia, of whom about half are still actively affected. At any one time there are about 40 000 individuals in UK mental hospitals with a diagnosed schizophrenic state and another 60 000–70 000 having day care or attending outpatient clinics.

First admission rates for schizophrenia have dropped some 30% since the early 1960s as a result of changes in diagnostic and admission practices. The advent of new drugs and patterns of care in the 1950s led to a realization that for many people the long-term effects of schizophrenia need not be as severe or as enduring as was once feared. Today, half of those diagnosed as suffering from schizophrenia recover; this is in dramatic contrast to four or five decades ago when entry into a mental hospital with such illness usually led to long-term incarceration in an institutional environment.

The chance of being diagnosed as schizophrenic is between two and three times greater in America than it is in Britain, but studies based on the use of a standardized diagnostic interview have shown that there is no underlying difference in the incidence of the disease in the two countries. Rather, it is apparent that American psychiatrists tend to regard as schizophrenia those conditions which in Britain would be diagnosed as affective disorders.

The prevalence of schizophrenia is highest in inner city areas and it was at one time thought that the poverty and social isolation of these localities were aetiological factors. Subsequent studies have shown that it is movement into such areas, either because the indivduals are seeking isolation or because they tend to be rejected by more structured communities less tolerant of deviance, which results in the concentration of such cases. In Sweden, it has been found that the prevalence of schizophrenia in the north of the country is some three times that existing in the less harsh and less isolated parts of Scandanavia. One explanation is that people less temperamentally suited to living with relatively low levels of social contact tend to move away faster than do those with withdrawn schizoid personalities. In Eire, schizophrenia rates appear to be high — both absolutely (especially in the isolated west) and relative to rates amongst Irish immigrants to England.

There is a clear positive correlation between low social class and the incidence of diagnosed schizophrenia. A causal realtionship was once suspected but subsequent research has revealed high levels of downward social mobility among schizophrenic people. The fathers of schizophrenics do not show any social class preponderance. Schizophrenia usually becomes apparent early in life, the highest incidence being among men in their twenties. In women, rates are a little lower and the average age of onset rather later, particularly in the case of paranoid schizophrenia.

The incidence is up to 40% higher in children where both parents are affected. But 90% of people who have a parent, brother, sister or child diagnosed as schizophrenic do not themselves develop the condition, at least as an overtly recognized psychiatric abnormality.

Twin studies have provided evidence of the importance of heredity in schizophrenia and some authorities have postulated that it is recessively inherited. Studies of environmental influences in schizophrenia have so far proved inconclusive.

Prevention

There are at present no known preventive measures for those at risk of developing schizophrenia.

PSYCHOPATHIC STATES

These are persistent disorders of the mind (whether or not accompanied by subnormality of intelligence) which result in abnormally aggressive or seriously irresponsible conduct on the part of the patients.

Epidemiology

There is no specific cause, but a social factor which stands out pre-eminently in a large number of psychopathic cases is a history of a broken home or illegitimacy. In a small number of male criminal psychopaths, a chromosomal abnormality (an extra Y chromosome) has been found.

Prevention

There are no known preventive measures.

ALCOHOL DEPENDENCE SYNDROME

This is a state, psychic and usually also physical, resulting from taking alcohol, characterized by behavioural and other responses that always include a compulsion to take alcohol on a continuous or periodic basis in order to experience its psychic effects and sometimes to avoid the discomfort of its absence. Tolerance may or may not be present. The characteristic of this syndrome is addiction to alcohol and it is to be distinguished from 'alcohol related disabilities' which are the mental, physical or social harm associated with drinking. Often the two states coexist. When the word 'alcoholism' is used here, it refers to the dependence syndrome.

Epidemiology

There has been a rising trend in alcohol cosumption since 1945 and this has been closely matched by hospital admissions for alcoholism and deaths from cirrhosis. In recent years there has been a significant rise in female drinking. The prevalence of alcoholism in a country is related to average alcohol intake per head; a rise in overall consumption increases the number of heavy drinkers and the number of alcohol-related problems.

The highest consumption of alcohol tends to be among young, unmarried, separated or divorced males. Many factors influence the intake of alcohol. These include the price of alcoholic beverages, licensing restrictions on their sale, cultural attitudes to alcohol consumption and drunkenness, the opportunities for drinking and pressures to do so. Although the total consumption of alcohol is similar in all social classes, middle-class people tend to drink more frequently but less heavily — and more often wine and spirits. Working-class people drink more heavily — and especially beer. Certain occupations — including journalists, doctors, publicans and people in entertainment — are particularly at risk. Important socioeconomic factors that lead to alcohol abuse are unemployment, a competitive and stressful lifestyle, depression and a fall in the real cost of alcoholic drinks.

Estimates of the number of alcoholics are unsatisfactory because of the lack of a suitable definition, difficulties of establishing danger levels of alcohol intake and the formidable problems of carrying out surveys. One such survey uncovered less than half the known alcohol consumption. It has been estimated that there are approximately half a million people in England and Wales with a serious drinking problem, of whom 150 000 are alcohol dependants. It is thought that about 8% of the total adult population are heavy drinkers, 2% problem drinkers and 0.4 per cent alcohol dependent. The number admitted for hospital treatment in any one year is about 20 000, and those identified in general practice in the order of 40 000 or more. Eight per cent of the population (3 million individuals) are thought to be drinking sufficient to show detectable biochemical abnormalities.

Men with alcohol problems at one time outnumbered women by roughly five to one, but the sex ratio is lessening (it is now 2:1) as a result of more women drinking regularly.

Studies have repeatedly shown that rates of dependence are considerably raised among those with an alcohol-dependent parent. While genetic factors may account for this, social factors cannot be excluded. Boys tend from an early age to be encouraged to drink more than girls, and children tend to follow their parents' drinking patterns. Twin, adoption and family studies of alcohol addiction have produced conflicting results. Overall mortality among alcoholics is twice the expected level and, for women aged 15–39, it has been shown to be 17 times the expected rate. Whereas only about 3000 death certificates a year mention alcohol, the true premature mortality linked to drinking is more probably in the order of at least 5000–10 000 per annum. The suicide rate may be as much as 70 times that of the general population.

Prevention

Measures that have been suggested for reducing the intake of alcohol are: the education of young people concerning the damage which alcohol can inflict upon their health and the danger that even comparatively small quantities can affect judgement, an increase in its cost (although this might cause additional harm to the most socially deprived sections of society if spending on essentials were cut), a reduction in the number of places where alcohol can be purchased, a ban on drink advertising and changing the attitudes of society to alcohol. Also important is the need to provide help for problem drinkers and alcohol dependents, either by voluntary organizations (such as Alcoholics Anonymous and the National Council on Alcoholism) or through specialized centres for the treatment of alcoholism.

General practitioners often fail to recognize alcohol problems in their patients, tending instead to diagnose coexisting conditions like anxiety and depression. The workplace can provide a good setting for preventive intervention and the encouragement of problem drinkers to seek help.

OTHER FORMS OF DRUG DEPENDENCE

Among the dependence-producing drugs are: barbiturates, benzodiazepines, amphetamines, cannabis, cocaine, hallucinogens, morphine-type drugs (morphine, heroin, codeine, and synthetic drugs having morphine-like effects such as methadone and pethidine), inhalants and volatile solvents. Dependence is a state characterized by a compulsion to take the drug on a continuous or periodic basis in order to experience its mental effects, and sometimes to avoid the discomfort of its absence.

Epidemiology

Some of these drugs, like cannabis and opium, have been used for centuries. In Europe and the USA in the last century opiates were often taken in the form of medicines and social concern led to legislation to restrict their use to situations where they were medically necessary and to be available only on prescription. The rise in illicit drug consumption that occurred in many countries during the 1960s was checked temporarily, and then disturbing reports appeared of a growing prevalence of heroin consumption in Western Europe, including Britain. The prevalence of drug misuse and dependence is even more difficult to assess than for alcohol, because their consumption is often illicit. Calculations based on the number of patients attending clinics for prescription of morphine-like drugs are acknowledged to be an underestimate of the problem. A report in 1982 suggested that there might be 40 000 people in Britain with serious drug problems but by 1986 this had probably risen to 500 000. Surveys have shown that cannabis preparations are the most widely used; amphetamines, barbiturates and hallucinogens are next in popularity; morphine-type drugs are those used least.

Evidence for an inborn tendency to addiction is much less than for dependence on alcohol. Drug use by friends and acquaintances is an important determinant; during adolescence especially, the need to conform to the behaviour of one's peers is often strong. Illicit drug use has been described as a kind of communicable disease which spreads from user to user. Peer pressures and the boredom of an isolated existence seem to encourage experimentation, with continued use of a drug as an escape from tedium.

Personality studies of illicit drug users show that, compared with non-users, they are more neurotic and anxious and are more likely to have an unhappy home and school life. It seems likely that most of them have emotional disturbances that antedate their contact with drugs. The neurotic may indulge to relieve tension, the psychopath to get a thrill and the psychotic to alleviate depression or suppress delusions. A study of the families of drug dependent adolescents has shown a high prevalence of psychiatric illness among the parents, usually in the form of alcoholism in the fathers and depressive illness in the mothers. There are also those patients who have become addicted to drugs induced through their legitimate use during medical treatment. Many thousands in this country are dependent on hypnotics or minor tranquillizers prescribed by their doctors.

The availability of drugs is another important factor. A major epidemic of amphetamine abuse occurred in Japan immediately following the Second World War and was traced directly to the release for sale to the public of large stores of surplus methamphetamine. It involved more than a million people and it is remarkable that it occurred in a population which until then had been relatively free of all types of drug abuse. There were also alarming reports of addiction among American forces in Vietnam where drugs were readily available and cheap. The availability of drugs to doctors and nurses has sometimes led to abuse by members of these professions. The incidence of dependence in Britain has fallen as a result of the campaign to reduce the prescribing of amphetamines.

Although dependence on drugs leads to criminal offences involving illegal possession or supply of drugs, as well as theft to obtain drugs or the money to exchange for drugs, surveys have shown that a considerable proportion incur minor convictions *before* they become implicated with drug consumption. For example, more than half of those identified as heroin addicts have a history of delinquent behaviour or a criminal conviction before they first use heroin.

Drug dependence, especially on opiates, lowers life expectancy but there is at present a paucity of adequate studies on the results of treatment. Improvement is related to the degree of social integration that the user has established or preserved. A satisfactory outcome is favoured by sustained contact with relatives and with acquaintances who do not use drugs, and by having employment. The development of abstinence from drugs is generally associated with improvement in other psychosocial spheres of adjustment, but this is not invariable and some abstinent people remain unemployed, are psychologically distressed, or have difficulties with interpersonal relationships. There is a tendency for opioid-dependent persons to mature out of drug usage and approximately 40% are abstinent by the end of 10 years.

Prevention

The development of rapid means of transport has contributed to the growth of international associations organized for illegal drug running. An international system of drug control is, therefore, essential and much is being done by United Nations agencies and other international bodies. There must be severe penalties for those involved in drug trafficking and adequate resources for their detection.

Educational programmes have so far not been demonstrated to be very effective. Studies have shown only minor and often transitory changes in the knowledge and attitudes of recipients; important alterations in behaviour are rarely demonstrated. Nevertheless, we believe that there is an important role for education aimed at policy makers and those concerned with law enforcement. The public needs to be informed of the dangers that arise from the use of drugs, and facilities must be available to advise parents and counsel drug takers.

In Britain, medical practitioners are forbidden to prescribe heroin, dipipanone or codeine to a drug-dependent person. They are also obliged to notify the Chief Medical Officer of the Home Office of any person whom the doctor considers, or has reasonable grounds to suspect, is addicted to certain controlled drugs.

SUICIDE AND PARASUICIDE

These are deliberate acts, whether physical, drug overdosage or poisoning, done in the knowledge that they are potentially lethal and, in the case of drug overdosage, that the amount taken is excessive. When the act is not fatal, it is referred to as 'parasuicide' or 'deliberate self-harm'.

Epidemiology

Each year in England and Wales, approximately 4000 people take their own lives. This is equivalent to slightly less than 20% of all unnatural deaths and 0.7% of mortality from all causes. However, among deaths in the age group 25–29 years, the latter proportion rises to 12%. These figures undoubtedly underestimate the true incidence of suicide but to what extent remains unclear.

Suicides among both sexes decreased significantly during the two World Wars; the female rate in 1915 was the lowest experienced so far this century. This association may in part be attributed to a greater degree of social integration at such times and the attainment of very high levels of employment. Peaks have coincided with years of economic depression in Britain, but it would be misleading to postulate a causal relationship between unemployment and the suicide rate.

The decline in suicides in the 1960s (which was unique to England and Wales) has been attributed to improved knowledge and treatment of psychiatric illness, the introduction of routine psychiatric consultation following attempted suicide, the steady improvement in emergency services and hospital treatment of poisoning, the rapid growth of the Samaritans, the introduction from 1958 onwards of natural gas which is virtually free of carbon monoxide (which was accompanied by a rapid fall in suicides due to domestic gas), and a fall in barbiturate prescribing.

Throughout the whole of this century male suicide rates have remained substantially higher than female rates. Since the late 1950s the older groups, both males and females, have experienced a consistent fall in the incidence of suicide. Suicide rates increase rapidly up to age 45, then rise more slowly (see Fig. 14.1) and reach a peak in the age range 75–84 years. About 20% of suicides now occur in people over the age of 60.

Poisoning is the major single cause of suicide, accounting for 40% of such deaths in males and 60% in females. Hanging and strangulation are the next leading cause, accounting for approximately 30% of suicide deaths in males and 20% in females. Suicide rates are particularly high in social class V (SMR 184) and they correlate with social isolation and social mobility.

Almost all completed suicides have a history of mental illness, notably depression and/or chronic alcoholism. In London, the boroughs with the highest rates contain a large proportion of people who have changed their residence within a year of the last census, many single-person households and a low incidence of marriage. It is suggested that these findings support the hypothesis that people likely to kill themselves tend to concentrate in certain areas, rather than the alternative view that the social factors precipitating suicide are more common in certain boroughs than in others.

The prinicpal source of information on parasuicide is the Hospital In-patient Enquiry (HIPE) but such hospital-based information is likely to underestimate the extent of parasuicide because some patients are treated in short-stay wards which are not HIPE registered. Hospital data also ex-clude episodes of minor self-inflicted injury treated (without further referral) by general practitioners and cases in which no medical attention is sought. There has been an alarming increase in the number of episodes of poisoning each year; this contrasts with the trend for completed suicide which has tended to stabilize or even fall.

In England and Wales there are approximately 121 000 discharges and deaths each year related to poisonings; about 90% of these involve medicinal agents. A reasonable estimate of the current incidence of self-poisoning is probably in the region of 100 000 episodes per annum. On this basis it appears that there are at least 20 cases of parasuicide for every completed suicide.

The highest rates of parasuicide occur in the age group 20–24 years in males and 15–24 years in females; it is among young people that the highest rates of increase have occurred. At all pre-retirement ages, rates are sub-stantially higher in females and the long-term tendency is for male rates to fall and for female rates to rise.

Prevention

One of the most important prerequisites for reducing the incidence of suicide and parasuicide lies in the identification of individuals at risk. However, this is not an easy task. Many suicides occur 'suddenly' without any consultation for psychological problems in the few months before death, possibly because the patients perceive their general practitioner as being disapproving, unsym-pathetic, or too busy, or because they are unaware of available sources of help. But a number of investigations have shown that more than half of para-suicide patients and three-quarters of suicides are in medical contact shortly before their episode of self-harm or death. Considerable potential therefore exists for a substantial reduction in suicidal behaviour.

A large proportion of individuals who deliberately harm themselves do so with medicines that can be obtained only on prescription. Seventy percent of suicide patients communicate their ideas beforehand and 40% state their intention unequivocally. The general practitioner is the professional person most familiar with individual patient histories and is in a good position to monitor significant changes in circumstances as well as sudden risk-inducing events such as bereavement and other forms of loss. The reasons for the failure of general practitioners to avert the subsequent episodes are unclear. They could include the time pressures experienced in general practice, the prescription of psychotropic medicines as a ready solution, and the inability or reluctance of patients to identify and discuss the causes of their distress.

Most parasuicide patients admitted to hospital need supportive care, rather than active treatment, but there is conflicting evidence as to whether psychiatric care or social work after discharge help to prevent further suicide attempts.

DEMENTIA IN OLD AGE

Irreversible and usually progressive organic disease of the brain in old age is characterized clinically by failing memory, intellectual deterioration and behavioural disturbance. For the more severely affected, the outcome is almost invariably a shortened life expectancy and a steadily diminishing capacity to undertake simple everyday tasks, culminating eventually in an inability to survive without considerable assistance.

Epidemiology

This is arguably the most significant problem currently facing our health services; 10% of the population over 65 years are affected by the condition and about half of these have symptoms of a severe degree. The prevalence increases steadily with age until 80 years and thereafter it increases rapidly; over 80 more than one person in five is affected. The incidence rates for males and females do not differ significantly, confirming that the higher prevalence among females is a reflection of their longer survival. The dementia problem will become more acute throughout the remaining years of the present century as the number of persons over 80 increases. Increased mortality has been found both in hospital and in community samples of elderly patients with dementia.

No evidence has emerged implicating environmental influences such as isolation or poor social conditions. These factors are often found in association with senile dementia but appear to be a consequence of the condition rather than having a causal role.

The concordance rate for identical twins is 43% and for non-identical twins 8%. The risk of developing senile dementia is four times greater in the relatives of demented persons than in members of unaffected families. It is concluded that this increased risk reflects the influence of genetic factors.

Prevention

Dementia is due to a progressive degeneration of brain cells and, in our present state of knowledge, there are no known means of preventing this common condition.

Index

172